Blond, blonde (blond). *a.* and *sb.* Forms: 5 blounde, 7– blonde, 8– blond. [a. F. *blond,* blonde yellow-haired, 'a colour midway between golden and light chestnut' (Littré), = Sp. *blondo,* It. *biondo*:—med. L. *blondus, blundus* yellow (explained in a passage quoted by Du Cange '*flavus* qui vulgo dicitur *blondus*'). Origin uncertain: see Diez and Littré. In English used by Caxton (in form *blounde*); reintroduced from mod. Fr. in 17th c., and still so far treated as French, as to be usually written with final *e* when applied to a woman, esp. substantively, *a blonde*; otherwise commonly written *blond* like the Fr. masculine.

A. *adj.* Properly (of the hair): Of a light golden brown, light auburn; but commonly used in sense of light-coloured, 'fair', as opposed to 'dark', or 'brunette', and extended to the complexion of those who have hair of this colour.

BLONDES
by Paula Yates

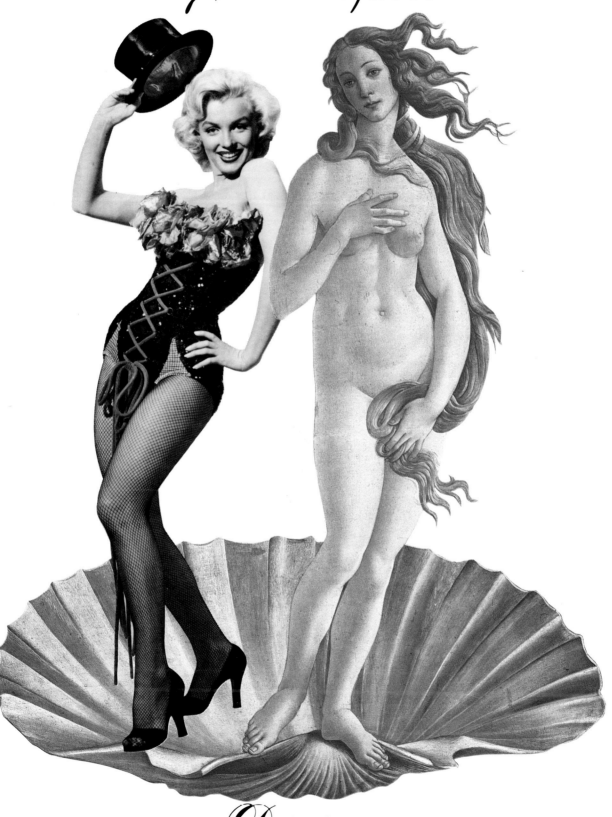

A *Delilah* BOOK
DISTRIBUTED BY THE PUTNAM PUBLISHING GROUP
N E W • Y O R K

To Chris and Carol.

A Delilah Book
Delilah Communications, Ltd.
118 East 25th Street
New York, N.Y. 10010

ISBN: 0-88715-001-2

First published in the United States of America by Delilah
Communications, Ltd. in 1984. Originally published in the
United Kingdom by Michael Joseph, Ltd. in 1983.

Designed by Bernard Higton.

Phototypeset by MS Filmsetting Ltd., Frome, Somerset,
England

Printed and bound in Italy by New Interlitho

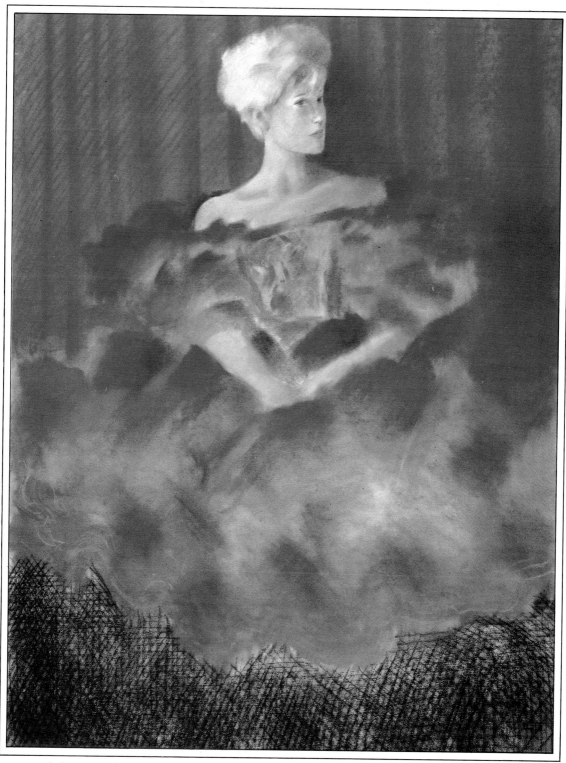

I have always wanted to be the sort of woman men kill for.
I have failed.
Others haven't.
This is their story.
They were all blondes.

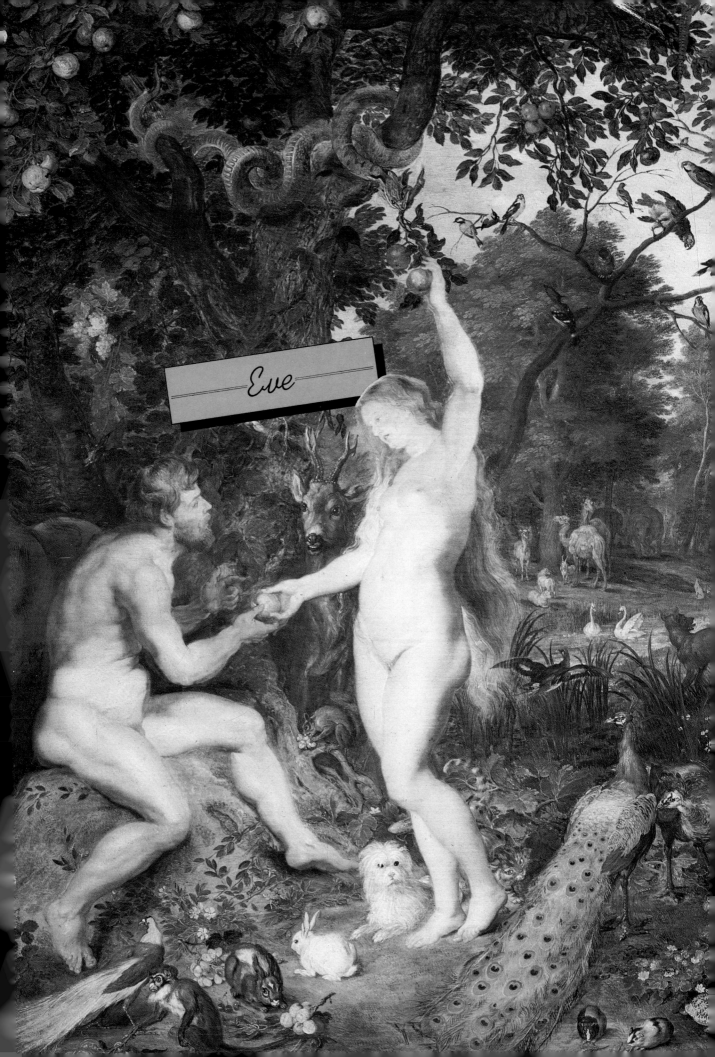

Eve

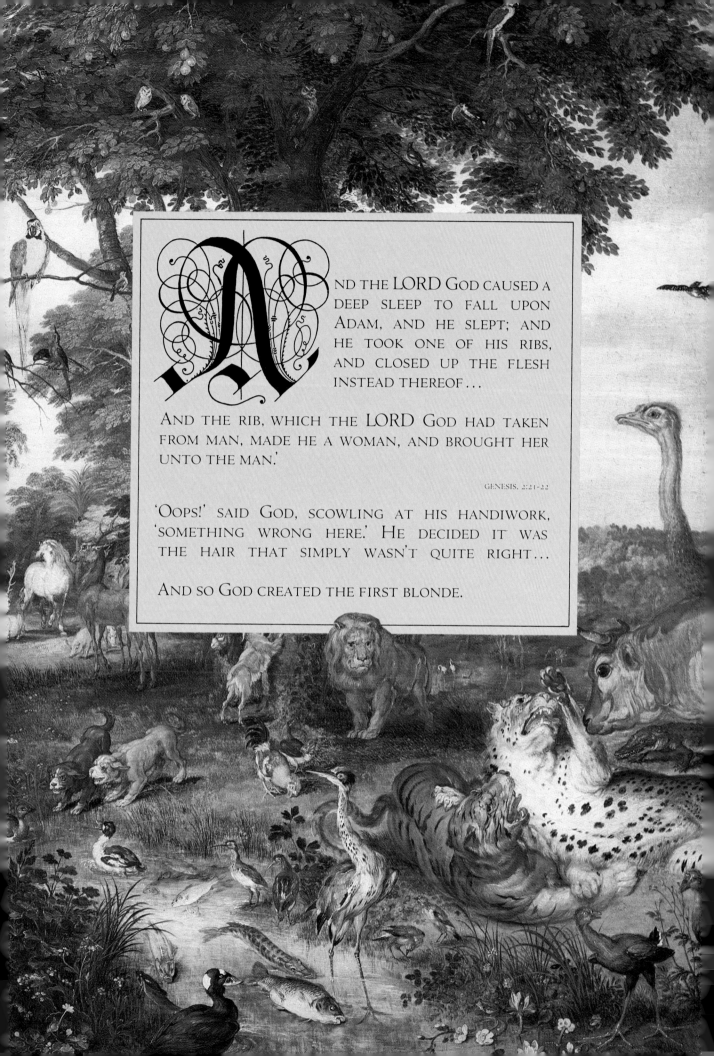

And the LORD God caused a deep sleep to fall upon Adam, and he slept; and he took one of his ribs, and closed up the flesh instead thereof...

And the rib, which the LORD God had taken from man, made he a woman, and brought her unto the man.'

GENESIS, 2:21-22

'Oops!' said God, scowling at his handiwork, 'something wrong here.' He decided it was the hair that simply wasn't quite right...

And so God created the first blonde.

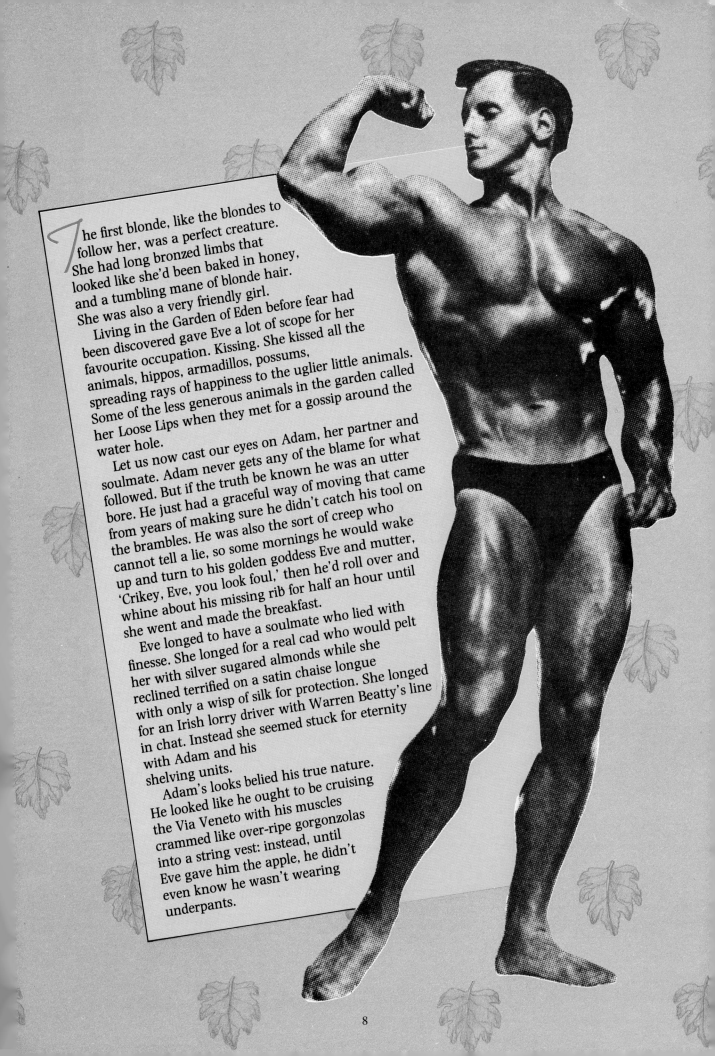

The first blonde, like the blondes to follow her, was a perfect creature. She had long bronzed limbs that looked like she'd been baked in honey, and a tumbling mane of blonde hair. She was also a very friendly girl.

Living in the Garden of Eden before fear had been discovered gave Eve a lot of scope for her favourite occupation. Kissing. She kissed all the animals, hippos, armadillos, possums, spreading rays of happiness to the uglier little animals. Some of the less generous animals in the garden called her Loose Lips when they met for a gossip around the water hole.

Let us now cast our eyes on Adam, her partner and soulmate. Adam never gets any of the blame for what followed. But if the truth be known he was an utter bore. He just had a graceful way of moving that came from years of making sure he didn't catch his tool on the brambles. He was also the sort of creep who cannot tell a lie, so some mornings he would wake up and turn to his golden goddess Eve and mutter, 'Crikey, Eve, you look foul,' then he'd roll over and whine about his missing rib for half an hour until she went and made the breakfast.

Eve longed to have a soulmate who lied with finesse. She longed for a real cad who would pelt her with silver sugared almonds while she reclined terrified on a satin chaise longue with only a wisp of silk for protection. She longed for an Irish lorry driver with Warren Beatty's line in chat. Instead she seemed stuck for eternity with Adam and his shelving units.

Adam's looks belied his true nature. He looked like he ought to be cruising the Via Veneto with his muscles crammed like over-ripe gorgonzolas into a string vest: instead, until Eve gave him the apple, he didn't even know he wasn't wearing underpants.

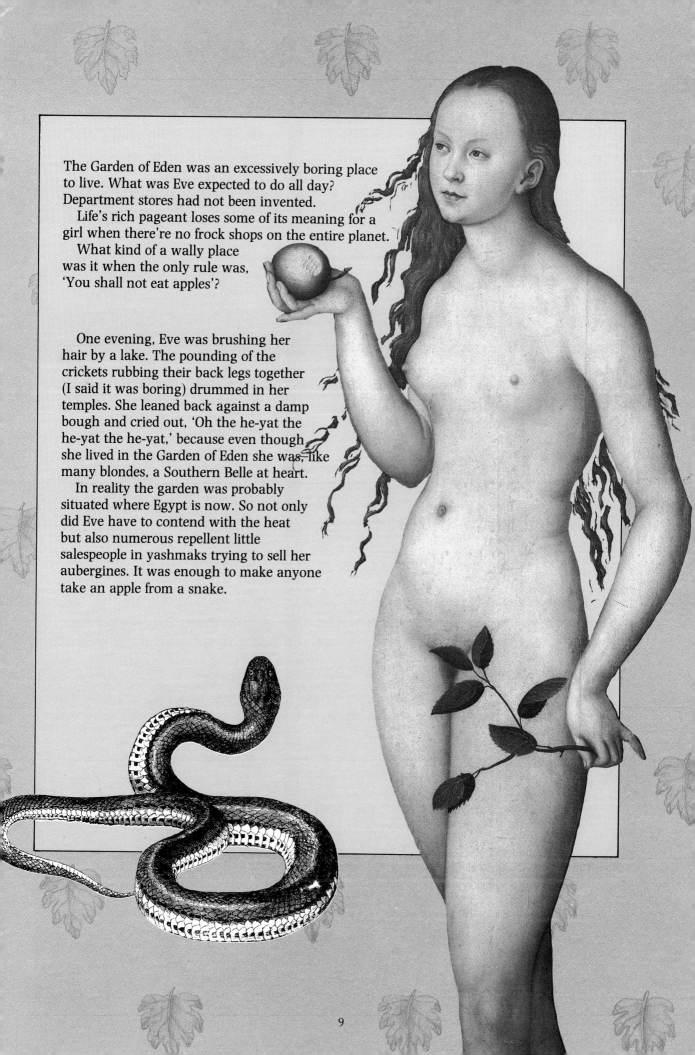

The Garden of Eden was an excessively boring place to live. What was Eve expected to do all day? Department stores had not been invented.

Life's rich pageant loses some of its meaning for a girl when there're no frock shops on the entire planet.

What kind of a wally place was it when the only rule was, 'You shall not eat apples'?

One evening, Eve was brushing her hair by a lake. The pounding of the crickets rubbing their back legs together (I said it was boring) drummed in her temples. She leaned back against a damp bough and cried out, 'Oh the he-yat the he-yat the he-yat,' because even though she lived in the Garden of Eden she was, like many blondes, a Southern Belle at heart.

In reality the garden was probably situated where Egypt is now. So not only did Eve have to contend with the heat but also numerous repellent little salespeople in yashmaks trying to sell her aubergines. It was enough to make anyone take an apple from a snake.

To a passing stranger Eve might have looked like a woman
on the verge of a severe asthma attack, but it was simply
boredom gripping her every blonde fibre.
And then she saw the snake . . .

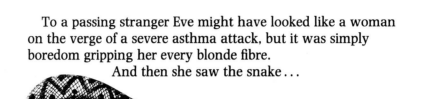

'Hellohisssssssssss,' said the snake,
'fansssssseeee a bit of thissss apple
big girl?'

'You know it's not allowed,' said Eve, but she
was not a girl who needed a lot of encouragement. 'What if I
do,' she said curiously, looking at the succulent red apple.

'If you do, you will realize you are naked and have to wear
clothes,' said the snake. 'But you will
alwaysssssssss be ssssssspecial becaussse
of your yellow hairr,' he informed her
helpfully . . .

This decided her. She gave the snake
a peck on what she imagined would
be the handle of a handbag in about
a week's time and bit the apple and
so did Adam who was taking a rest
from grouting the tiles.

And then the skies opened . . .

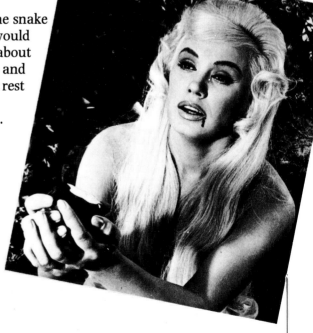

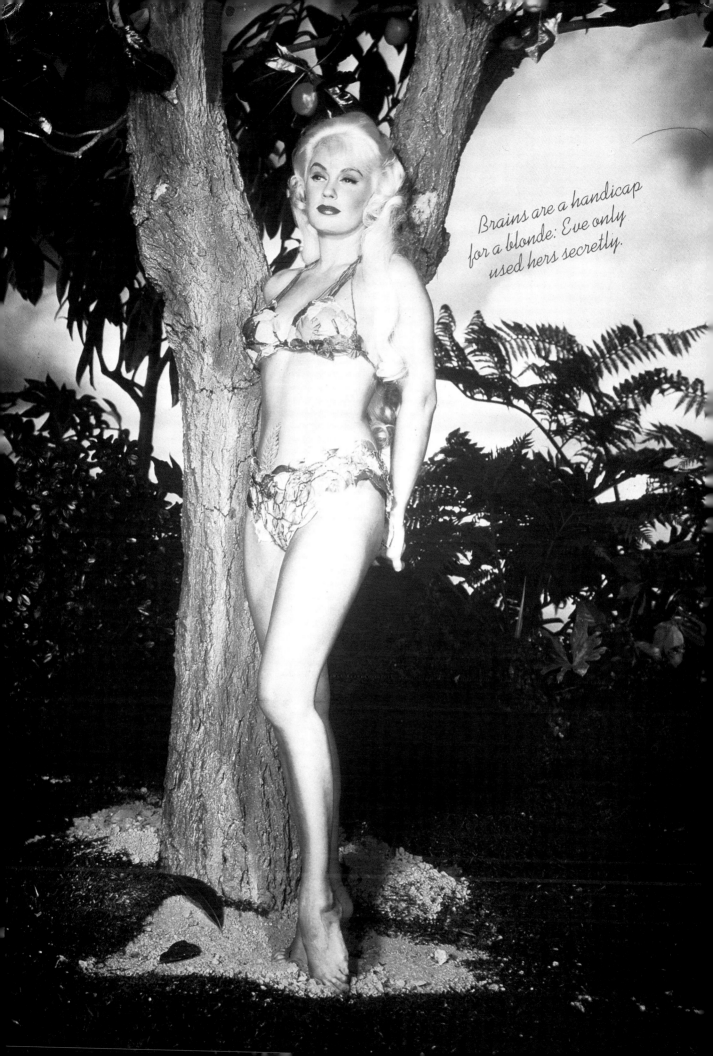

Brains are a handicap for a blonde: Eve only used hers secretly.

*W*ithout the blonde, Lord Clark would have had nothing to write about. Once they realized early in the dawn of civilization that blondes do indeed have more FUN, the pursuit of blonde hair became one of womankind's Great Aims. While men aspired to captivate a blonde, women aspired not to have two inches of black roots.

Blondes will always seem unthreatening to men, who continue to act as if the most determinedly calculating blonde will inevitably become a dizzy sex kitten, be putty in his hunky hand.

The blonde, of course, realized the minute she took the big step towards being a real pretend blonde that a whole world of blondeness opens up. A world of getting away with it...

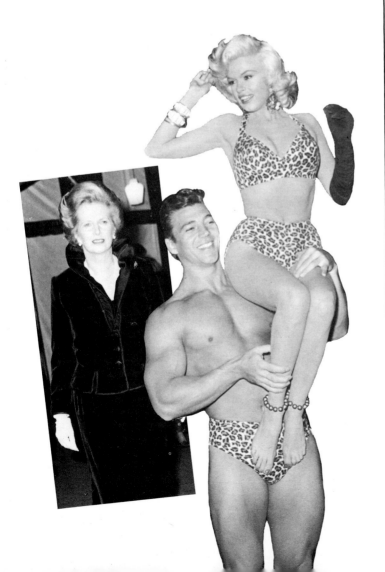

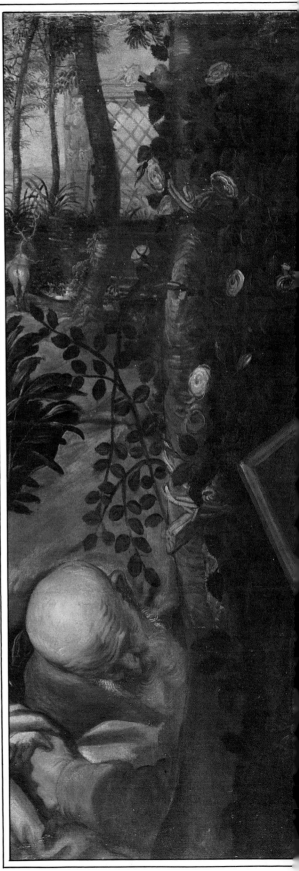

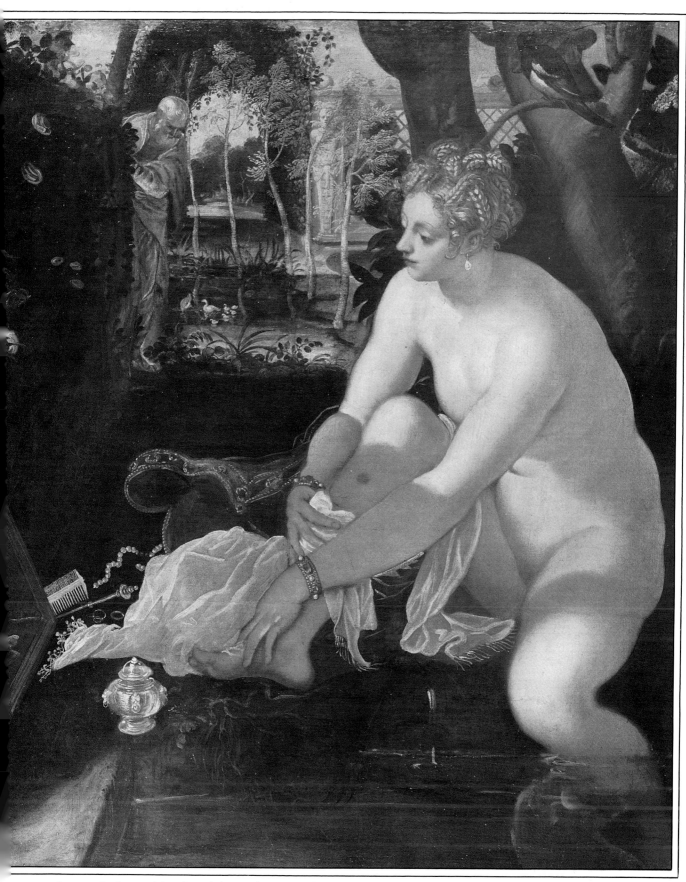

Eve, like all the blondes to follow her, was simply getting her priorities right . . . scent, security, poodles, adoration, clothes and the heady sense of power were all hers from now on.

londes appear in the earliest written records almost five thousand years ago in Egypt. In 3066 BC, Queen Nitocris was described as 'the noblest and most beautiful woman, fair in colour'. From this moment, literature has consistently striven to secure the blonde's image in the minds of men. When she's not being a sexpot, she is lightness, goodness, and saintliness: a scented, pampered creature to be possessed only by the rich and powerful.

The Egyptians were also the first women to suffer in order to become blondes. The pussycat was God in Ancient Egypt and so the ideal beauty of the day looks to the modern viewer something like a reject from the chorus-line of *Cats*. Women sat for hours in the baking sun with Nile mud spread liberally over their heads. This was thought to aid the bleaching process. It didn't work very well despite trojan efforts by everyone involved, and soon coloured wigs became popular with women wishing to create the blonde effect. The ladies then returned to their primary interests – fucking, eye make-up and cat shows.

After 1150 BC, even more extravagant hair became popular and red, green, violet and blue wigs could be seen around town. Blonde hair had temporarily been put on the shelf due to the amount of women collapsing with severe sunstroke.

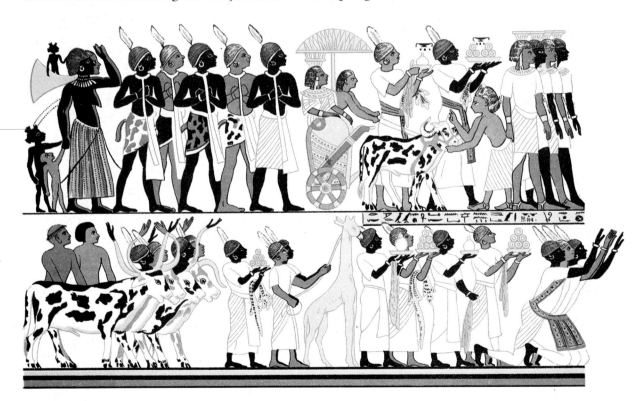

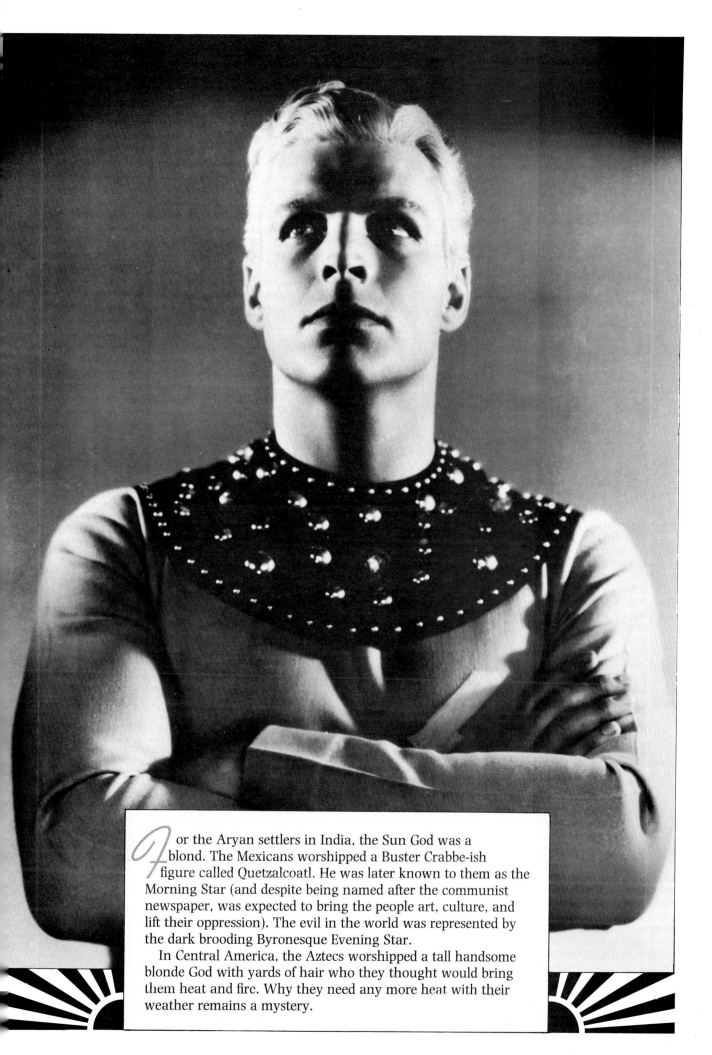

or the Aryan settlers in India, the Sun God was a blond. The Mexicans worshipped a Buster Crabbe-ish figure called Quetzalcoatl. He was later known to them as the Morning Star (and despite being named after the communist newspaper, was expected to bring the people art, culture, and lift their oppression). The evil in the world was represented by the dark brooding Byronesque Evening Star.

In Central America, the Aztecs worshipped a tall handsome blonde God with yards of hair who they thought would bring them heat and fire. Why they need any more heat with their weather remains a mystery.

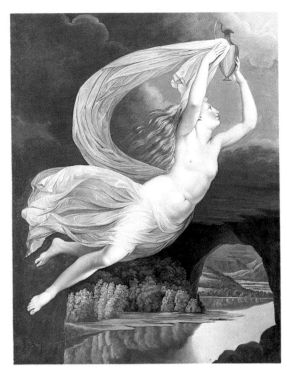

pounced on. Zeus was the best at it, turning himself into a swan or a bull or a sunbeam, depending on how he felt when he got up in the morning.

The three top blonde Goddesses – Aphrodite (Goddess of Love), Hera (Zeus' wife) and Athene (Goddess of Wisdom) – were always rowing about who was the prettiest. Olympus was like a pyjama party for Farrah, Cheryl and the poison dwarf.

Eventually they had to have a competition, judged by Paris, a square-jawed shepherd boy. Aphrodite won because she bribed him with the promise that he'd get the best blonde in the world.

So who did he marry? Helen of Troy, naturally.

Those Greeks started a whole trend in seeing the blonde as bad, decadent and tempting . . .

*A*ncient Greek mythology continued the tradition of fantasizing over big blonde heroes and heroines. Danae, the Mistress of Zeus, was so blonde that Zeus had to visit her in a shower of gold to get her to notice him at all.

The Ancient Greeks are greatly associated with blonde hair, a misconception that appears to stem almost entirely from Paul Newman's appearance in the *Silver Chalice*, in which he wore a shortie-style toga. The women of Greece were not often born blonde and were frequently mocked for their attempts at dyeing. Menander, a Greek poet of the fourth century, wrote, 'Now get out of this house, for no chaste woman should make her hair yellow', which seems a reasonable point. In Greece once a girl had blonde hair it was unlikely she'd remain chaste for more than ten minutes.

In the great Greek myths and legends, blondeness could get you anywhere and often did. Blondes were kidnapped (then again so was Tammy Wynette, but she talked so much that the kidnappers eventually couldn't stand it any longer and threw her out of the car). And they were

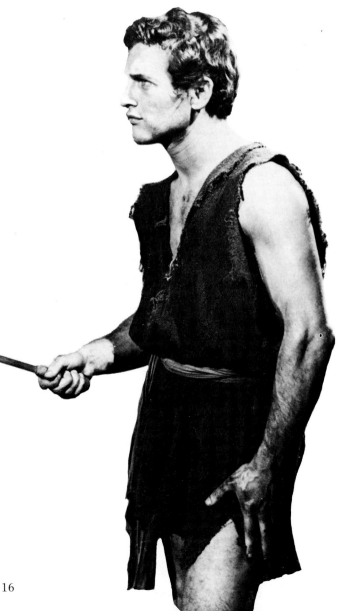

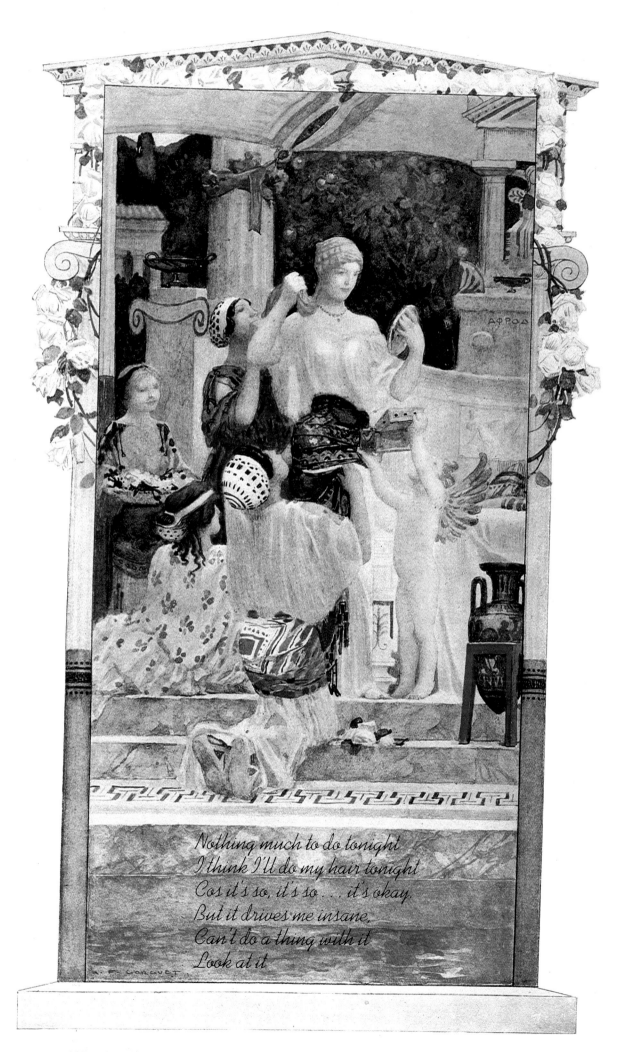

Nothing much to do tonight
I think I'll do my hair tonight
Cos it's so, it's so . . . it's okay.
But it drives me insane,
Can't do a thing with it
Look at it

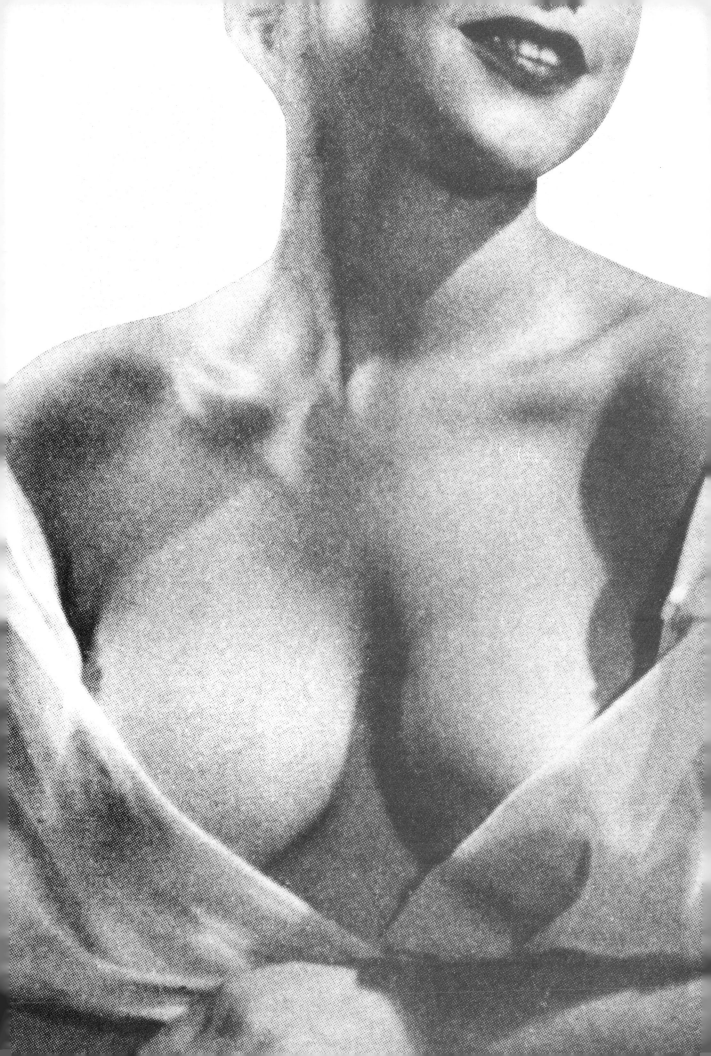

Helen was an exquisite beauty with lots of blonde hair, a voice like a lilting lute, a figure like a dream and soft red lips like a rose petal dipped in dew. Due to her extreme beauty she was also a little unlucky. A quick read through any Greek history book could leave one with the impression that there were few warriors, Gods, ducks, swans or kings who didn't at one point rape the poor girl. She was married several times, men captured her, ran away with her and sent wooden horses filled with soldiers to try and get her back home again. Quite apart from the battle of Troy, being married to Helen was a dangerous occupation. Her husbands were slain, maimed and made thoroughly miserable, plus Helen was always having children by all manner of punters depending on which book you read. But apart from being so lovely that men were willing to die for her, start wars for her and

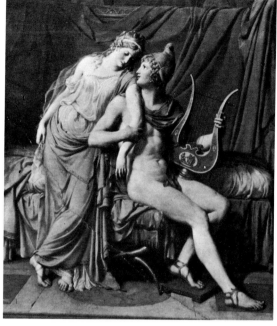

generally make fools of themselves, the thing that Helen was most famous for were her tits.

The beauty of Helen of Troy's chest was known throughout Greece. Songs were sung on mountainsides praising the beauty of the twin mounds. Helen, who was not as daft as one might imagine, knew the power of her bosom and regularly went without the protection of a liberty bodice. She often got them out and flashed them when the going got rough and those who viewed them seem to have been enslaved for life.

With this predilection for exposing herself in hot weather it is perhaps not surprising that so many interesting things happened to her. A scholar in the Little Ilaid – rather than the more famous Big Iliad – noted that 'Menelaos, when he somehow caught a glimpse of the breasts of naked Helen, threw away his sword.' Which seems to be the worst thing he could have done. Whenever Helen got her gear off trouble was inevitable.

Many legends refer to Helen as a 'deep-bosomed Okeanid'. But the paintings of Helen don't seem to do her justice. She doesn't look at all the sort of woman who stood on the prow of ships while the seas around her turned red from the blood of men dying because of her beauty. Let alone a girl whose mother did it with a swan . . .

Boadicea

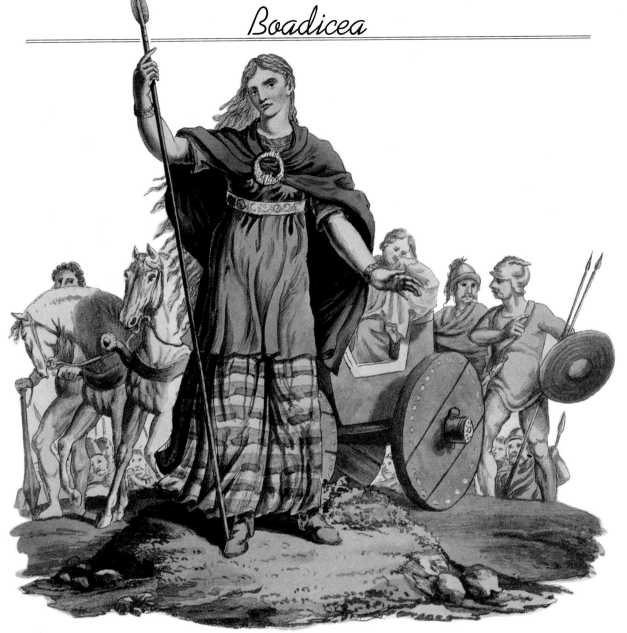

One of the first blondes in the proper history books is the British Queen, Boadicea. From descriptions, she might easily have been a man in drag, or just a large woman with severe premenstrual tension who led rampaging hordes through the country.

Living at a time when a tall man was about 5′ 2″, Boadicea was an Amazonian blonde with odd taste in clothes. She was like the Janet Street-Porter of the Northern Tribes. The strapping blonde with yard-long hair could be seen riding around wearing a long gold chain around her neck, a dress of many colours and an enormous golden brooch holding her cape in place. The Iceni, her people, were as fascinated then as *Women's Own* readers are now by every aspect of their royal family's life and often gossiped about the Queen, her clothes and her two daughters whom they doted upon. The people also worried about her terrible driving which was famous throughout the land: she would ride around like Ben Hur himself in her unsprung, brakeless carriage on the moors with two small children being flung fifteen feet in the air at every pot-hole and rabbit warren.

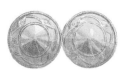

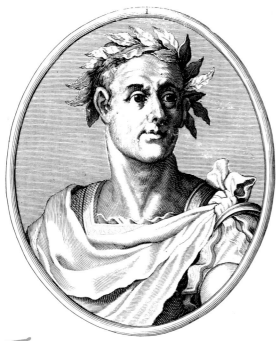

*T*hen Julius Caesar arrived.
Caesar felt that the British were a bunch of barbarians and nearly fainted from the smell of sheep droppings and laundry when he entered his first British home. He also reeled at the freezing cold draughts which wafted up his dress from day one. He was amazed to discover that wives in Britain were regarded as communal property, something that only referred to baths in Rome. And being something of a Roman version of McAlpine he couldn't believe that they still hadn't built proper roads, but with all the wife-sharing going on it's no wonder the Brits' minds were not running on road-building and hot-and-cold sewers.

The Romans were an entirely different race, of course, and arrived resplendent in their flimsy togas, with laurel wreaths and false gold beards, and set about building motorways. In between building roads they also imposed crippling taxes on the British, seizing their homes so that they would have somewhere to stay, while they were mosaicing their swimming pools. The Romans in fact had very similar taste in interior design to Diana Dors and the Raymond Revue Bar.

The final straw came when the Romans started using British children as slaves and cutting off their hair to send it back to make blonde wigs for their wives. That did it for big blonde Boadicea, who had no intention of going around bald in the northern winters. When news came that a Roman legion was marching towards the lands of the Iceni armed with swords and scissors she went totally ferocious.

Gathering her loyal followers together, Boadicea sacked Colchester, tossed the Ninth Roman Legion off the pier and threw their mosaic-decorated hairdressing implements into a ditch, where they were found in 1860 by a schoolteacher who was having an afternoon out with her divining rod. As the rabble grew bigger and bigger they destroyed settlements in London and St Albans. According to Tacitus, who retreated rapidly to the countryside, more than 70,000 Romans were killed during these bloody battles over the rates increases. They should have thought themselves lucky they didn't live in Lambeth.

Boadicea finally lost her control over the army who were nearly all killed in a Battle near Nuneaton. Not a very spectacular battle (Nuneaton hardly holds a place in military history along with Trafalgar and Waterloo), but Boadicea had already become synonymous with liberation from oppression and terror, and the fact she was a girl never entered into anyone's thinking. She took her place alongside the other great legends like Arthur and Camelot. A sort of Jane Fonda without the aerobics . . .

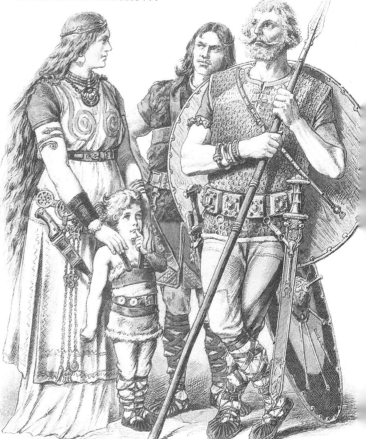

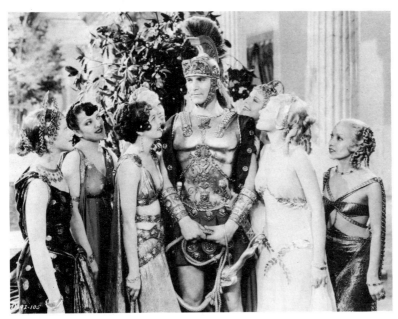

Pliny, this dye for fiery brunettes was a mixture of ground black beetles, leeches, and vinegar which was fermented for two months in a leaden vessel: it was so potent that if they swallowed it they'd have had black hair and matching teeth. Another problem for these women was that they could be smelled two miles away.

Galen, the medical treatise-writer, says that the main dye used for blondes was made from saffron which had to be scrubbed into the hair

*B*londes had got into their stride by Roman times. Dyeing wasn't quite the ludicrous performance it had been for the Egyptians and varying degrees of fairness could be achieved depending on how much time/money/bottle you had.

At first the only way to acquire the appearance of a Nordic floozy was to sprinkle your head liberally with gold dust. This was expensive. A little shake of the head would disperse a fortune on your shoulders like dandruff. This is perhaps the reason blondes have become associated with the sort of girls who can't say no. With gold dust on their heads it was more than they could afford to . . .

The wives of powerful men, who spent a lot of time and energy conquering weedier countries had easier access to fair hair. The long-suffering husbands would return from a long trip, to find their wingeing wives up to their necks in asses' milk being fanned by a nubile slave in a lamé loin-cloth – and present them with the hair of the conquered northern races. The wives upon receiving these gifts would leap out of the bath and make a huge fuss of the husbands.

There were other methods, of course – and it was far harder to become a sultry *dark*-haired temptress. Ladies would have to sit for hours with their mouth full of linseed oil, to prevent the dye trickling down their face and into their throats. Invented by

ferociously. In Italy the women were prepared to go to such lengths to go blonde that the local monks complained about the secret ointments they were using. One recipe instructed women to 'take dried cauls from the Orient and grind them into a powder, then mix with equal portions the yolks of eggs that have been boiled, and mix with wild honey. Rub onto the hair in the evening and wrap in a kerchief. Wash in the morning with olive-oil soap and fresh water.' Devotees then had to sit in direct sunlight and wait for the results. Other methods included bleaching the hair with elderberries, nutshells, vinegar sediment and plants. Men who were attracted ran the risk, if they attempted to run their hands through these silken locks, of having them trapped in a quagmire of boiled rabbits' bottoms, or actually severing them on the stiff bits, stuck together with leeches' droppings.

All this leads one to realize that blondes in

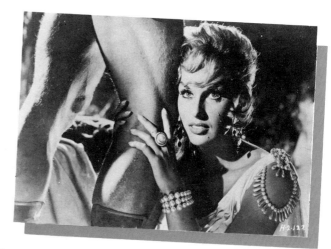

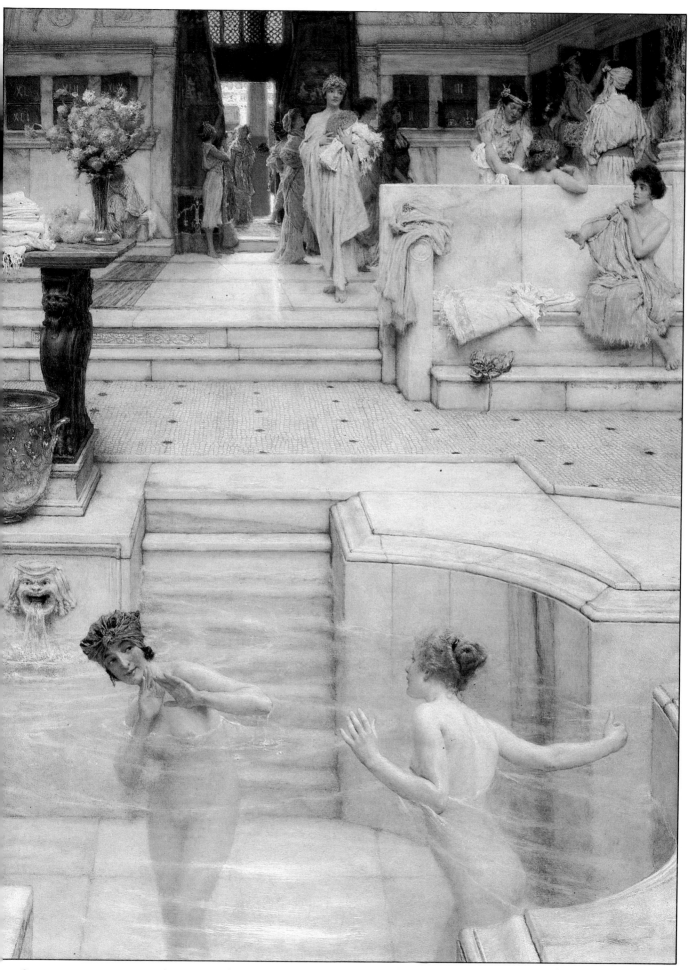

Roman women knew that a whole new world was open to the blonde:
a world of getting away with it without ever getting rumbled.

those days were rather smelly people, with not a lot of brain and quite a bit of sunstroke after a day in the broiling heat with their heads stuck through the veranda railings.

Nonetheless, it was in Roman times that the blonde became synonymous with the rampant hotsie. Prostitutes were not only taxed and provided with licences like Nevada, they were also required to wear blonde wigs as a mark of their profession. This regulation caused much confusion when 'blonde' wig-wearing Messalina, the notoriously unfaithful wife of Emperor Claudius, became a fashion leader. Many fat middle-aged ladies hoping to recapture their lost youth by emulating her antics must have found themselves getting offered a fiver by confused men.

Messalina

M essalina was something of a goer even by early Roman standards, where it was deemed perfectly acceptable to do it with lions, crocodiles and bears

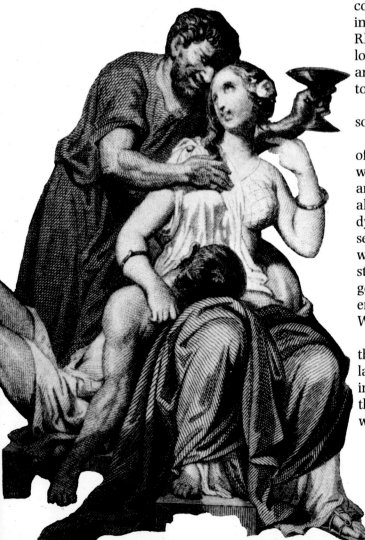

depending on who the Emperor was at the time. Messalina was the sort of girl who is after fun with a capital F, and was rumoured by the legions to be willing to get her laughing gear around anything available. On the quiet she kept nocturnal trysts with half the local builders and centurions, and their friends and relatives. Slipping off at the dead of night she would don an enormously flamboyant blonde wig which she was convinced was the perfect disguise. In fact, she couldn't have looked more conspicuous wandering around Rome in the middle of the night in her nightie and what appeared to be a blonde busby on hire from Bermans.

Her whole plan failed miserably time after time. After a torrid night of sin she would invariably forget to put her wig back on again and leave it slung under the bed. Her lovers would send the wig back to her by messenger the next morning. The arrival of her wig without her made her the source of much gossip around town. Less successful matrons in society boiled with jealousy. The poet Martial wrote of her: 'Her toilet table contains a thousand lies, and while she was in Rome her hair was blushing by the Rhine. A man was in no condition to say he loved her, for what he loved was not herself, and that which was herself was impossible to love.'

Which seems a little harsh. Messalina sounds like a game girl.

Reading Martial's comments on the ladies of the time it seems reasonable to suspect he was the sort of little poof given to hanging around the Dixie Peach hairdressing salon all day seeing who was having their hair dyed and who had their double chin sellotaped behind their ears and then writing poems about it. Despite him, women still felt that Messalina's great success with gentlemen was due entirely to the enchanting qualities of her blonde busby. Wig sales rapidly increased.

Ovid was another poetical super-grass of the day. He gleefully reported on a young lady he'd paid a visit to who was thrown into such a flurry by his unexpected arrival that she conducted their whole conversation with her wig on back to front.

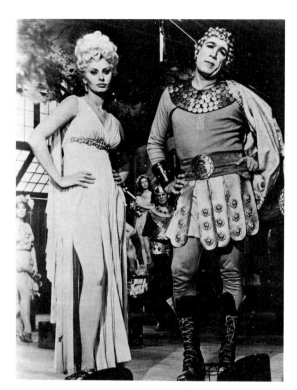

deformity: he suggests that Caesar always wore the laurel leaves to cover up his patchy bits. During the Imperial period of Rome, chunks of false hair were stuck onto the head to cover any bald patches.

Beards were an on-again off-again affair for most men. During the time of Cicero they were popular with young men, but frowned upon elsewhere. Marcus Livius wasn't allowed to take his seat in the Senate until he'd shaved his off. The Emperor Caligula, when he wasn't being wanked on from a dizzy height by nubile slaves from the East, wore a small stuck-on gold beard right on the end of his chin. He must have looked a real prawn.

From my extensive research into the entire history of the world it must be said that the Roman men were a bunch of girls' blouses – in fact they wore girls' skirts, leather ones – gossiping all day and trying to get their hands on the builders from the Colosseum site. Roman men spent large amounts of time perfuming and crimping their hair. Even athletes and great warriors worried about their barnets. Ovid says baldness was considered to be a terrible

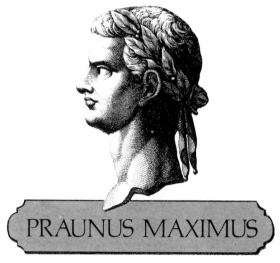

PRAUNUS MAXIMUS

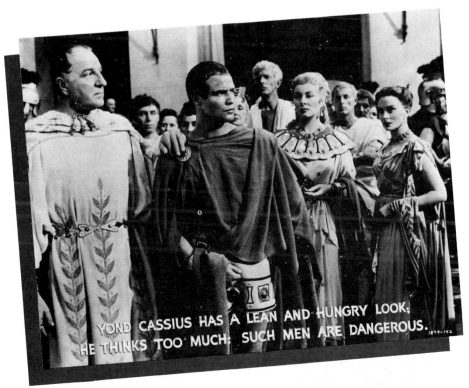

YOND CASSIUS HAS A LEAN AND HUNGRY LOOK. HE THINKS TOO MUCH; SUCH MEN ARE DANGEROUS.

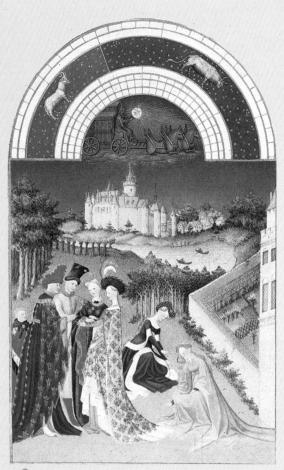

It is now revealed that the Courtly Love Conventions of the Middle Ages were not at all like the conventions of today. Far from being large gatherings of mushroom salesmen meeting at the Fontainbleu in Miami, they were dictates placed upon the knights of the day and the beautiful young women they dreamed of possessing. Needless to say in Mediaeval England the knights made sure that they almost always pined for another man's wife, removing any chance of them being expected to haul their armour up the aisle. They would gaze upon their fair maiden from afar, send her letters and poems, wear her colours at jousting matches and do things like fixing the tapestries when they fell down. In return she would simply inspire him to higher things and give him plenty of rivals to joust with, which of course was really the whole object of the exercise.

During the Middle Ages, hairstyles were even more exaggerated than they had become in Roman times when women spent all their money on solid gold cones to hold everything in the air. Women who did not possess enough money for an extensive retinue of servants were never seen before four o'clock in the afternoon. They spent hours in their bedrooms tussling with their hair-dos and crying, because at that rate no knight would ever spot them perusing the rose garden. Hair had to be pinned, curled, rolled around fat pads of stuffing and studded with precious stones.

The word 'blonde' was not much used. More common in poems of the time are descriptions like 'golden wire' – which is what it must have felt like after all they'd done to get it blonded.

The Mediaeval English author was very definite about his ideal heroine: blue eyes would sparkle, cheeks would be white or rose red, foreheads broad. She was required to have a good set of teeth, red lips like rose petals and of course blonde hair.

By contrast, Byzantine society, a late-flourishing Eastern offshoot of the Roman Empire, had a rather Californian view of the blonde. Byzantine blondes didn't exactly have forty-three-inch chests encased in apple-green fluorescent singlets and satin shorts, and didn't use the roller-skate as their sole form of transport from A to B, but they did share a similarly basic attitude to blondeness. It was associated by the Byzantine mind with strength, beauty and purity. Their theories on blondeness and its sexual potency sound like a back issue of *Health and Efficiency*. Byzantine blondes, had they not been so dignified and po-faced, would have been pictured in the twentieth century bounding around on topless beaches chasing multi-coloured balls.

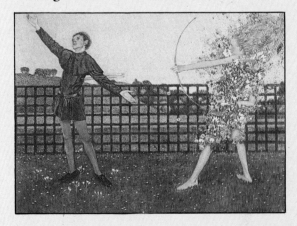

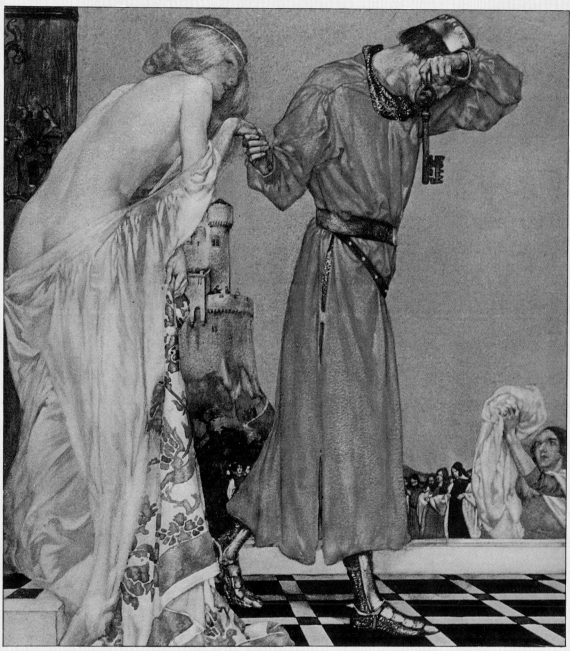

Lancelot comforts a dolorous lady by acting out scenes from 'A Streetcar Named Desire'.

The Mediaeval mind had by now decided that beauty was an outward sign of great goodness and purity. Ugliness was its obvious opposite. Romances of the time are littered with damsels in distress being rescued by tall handsome knights whose blond curls tumble out of their helmets as they lift their visors to kiss them. The knights all had piercing blue gazes and bronzed bodies like Gods ... which seems unlikely with our weather. Wickedness and evil were represented in these tales by horribly deformed giants or dwarf with long dirty sooty black beards. The beautiful knight was the perfect contrast with fair smooth skin and golden hair like a child's.

The tales of Camelot and Lancelot make one realize that despite the fact they didn't have loos, or dentists, and used sheep in their drawing rooms instead of storage heaters, the people of the dark ages were an intensely romantic bunch ...

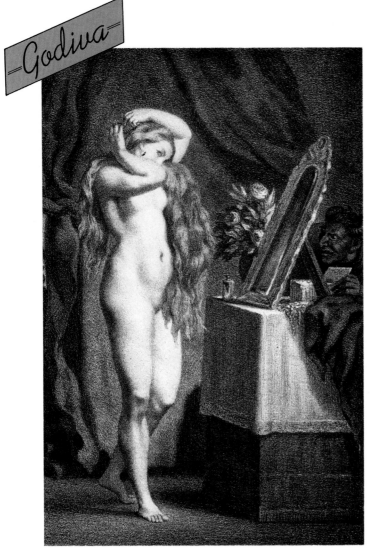

Godiva

the taxes. In the end he was so fed up with her wittering on that he forbade her to mention the subject. Didn't she realize that it was these taxes that were paying for her weekly trips to London and the stained-glass windows they'd just installed?

Nowadays what happened next would have caused a bunch of revolting hacks to descend upon Coventry, offering everyone a fiver for their side of the story and dressing up as striped roadworkers' tents in order to get sneak photos. In fact, the story was written up by the local monks, who must have suffered the fires of hell in their efforts not to become inflamed by the whole tale.

Matthew Paris elaborated the story in his *Chronica Majora* in the thirteenth century:

> The saintly countess, desiring to free the town from its burdensome and shameful servitude, often besought the Earl, her husband, to free the town from this slavery. She exasperated her husband with her unceasing request and extorted from him the following reply. 'Mount your horse naked,' he said, 'and ride through the marketplace of the town, from one side right to the other, while the people are congregated, and when you return you shall claim what you desire.' ... Then the Countess Godiva, beloved of God, on a certain day as it is said, mounting her horse naked, loosed her hair from its bands and her whole body was veiled except her fair white legs. Her journey unseen by a soul she returned rejoicing to her husband who counted it a miracle. Then Earl Leofric granted a charter freeing the city from its servitude and confirmed it with his seal ...

*A*round this time came the first example of a blonde utilizing her immense sexuality and her power over her husband in order to GET THINGS DONE ... Godiva could have been regarded as a sort of chesty social worker with unusual tactics, when she got the tax reform for Coventry simply by riding naked through the local market.

Godiva's husband, Earl Leofric, simply wanted to go about his business like any other eleventh-century British politician, despoiling church lands and inflicting huge taxes upon the people of Coventry, who were almost starving while coins chinked into his doublet. His saintly wife, for there was nothing bad ever said about Godiva, was busily trying to convince him to lift all

The only person to emerge from this story as fairly normal is Peeping Tom. According to the legends, which appear to have been written out by typesetters on a day off from the *Guardian*, Tom was a tailor's assistant.

While the rest of Coventry crouched nobly on their bedroom floors, praying for Godiva, Tom was rolling

28

around on his bedroom floor in an agony of indecision. In the end he heard her horse's hooves approaching and could not resist having a quick look. Unluckily for him, his window creaked and she caught him looking at her.

One can almost hear him the next day telling all his customers about her cellulite. 'Well, daahling, no *wonder* she didn't want anyone to have a peek!'

Godiva got her revenge, albeit a benevolent one. She decreed that henceforth young Tom always be referred to as Peeping Tom of Coventry. Which is a pretty good name for any new dress designer to have.

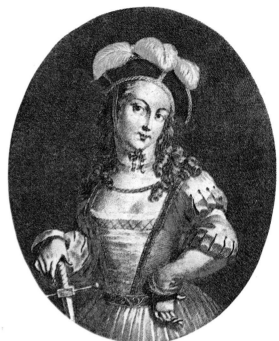

Joan of Arc — a girl who meant to set the world alight, but got her fingers burnt.

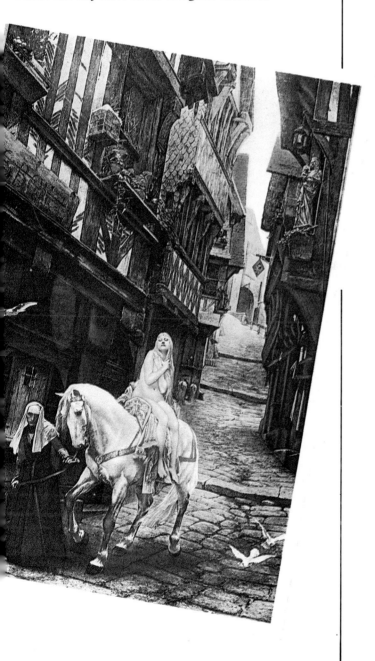

The Blonde strikes back

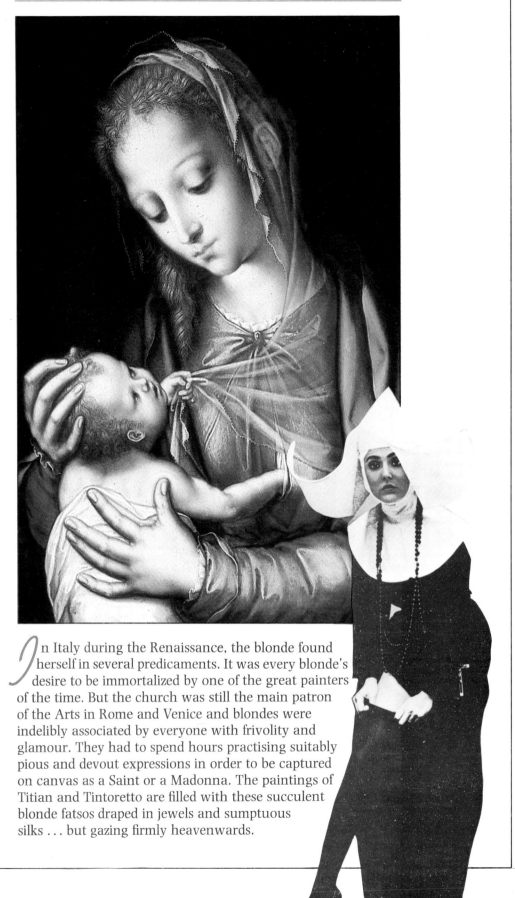

*I*n Italy during the Renaissance, the blonde found
herself in several predicaments. It was every blonde's
desire to be immortalized by one of the great painters
of the time. But the church was still the main patron
of the Arts in Rome and Venice and blondes were
indelibly associated by everyone with frivolity and
glamour. They had to spend hours practising suitably
pious and devout expressions in order to be captured
on canvas as a Saint or a Madonna. The paintings of
Titian and Tintoretto are filled with these succulent
blonde fatsos draped in jewels and sumptuous
silks . . . but gazing firmly heavenwards.

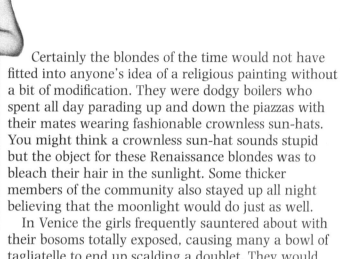

Certainly the blondes of the time would not have fitted into anyone's idea of a religious painting without a bit of modification. They were dodgy boilers who spent all day parading up and down the piazzas with their mates wearing fashionable crownless sun-hats. You might think a crownless sun-hat sounds stupid but the object for these Renaissance blondes was to bleach their hair in the sunlight. Some thicker members of the community also stayed up all night believing that the moonlight would do just as well.

In Venice the girls frequently sauntered about with their bosoms totally exposed, causing many a bowl of tagliatelle to end up scalding a doublet. They would add a sheer veil of rosy rouge to their chests for added effect. In the end the extravagances of the blonde community grew so uncontrolled that laws were actually passed to prevent further excesses of ostentatious behaviour. The Doge's daughters were the only women exempt from these bans on frilly underwear, various fabrics and some forms of jewellery.

On one occasion the Doge's blonde and beautiful niece sallied forth to a local fête wearing a dress made entirely out of cloth-of-gold, which does seem a little much for midday. Upon arrival she was sent straight home to change, and told that she knew perfectly well that ladies were only permitted to wear gowns with *sleeves* in this material.

*B*londe was everything. Firenzuolo was writing in his beauty book that in order to be ravishing a woman must have hair 'ranging from gold to honey' and then 'the colour of sunshine' – neither of which was easy if you happened to be a typical Latin spitfire with black hairy arms and a moustache to match . . .

Many different hair dyes were now available, in shades from golden or tawny to stripey, smoky and brilliant. The range was like the tom cats at the Chelsea cat show.

But looking at the dye recipes of the day, there seems to be no rhyme or reason why they should have been expected to make one blonde. Stinky ingredients like alum, black sulphur and honey were ladled onto numerous heads and then laid out to bake.

With that sort of pungent aroma rising in the heat, not much else was likely to get laid.

It was probably the appalling sexual frustration of these women, who looked like blonde Venuses but smelled like polecats, that led to the increasingly frenzied artistic activity found during this period in Italy. (One of the reasons so many women ended up being painted onto ceilings was the artist's desperate need to get as far away as possible from the smell.) Painters, architects, poets would sit on their balconies at a safe distance from their Muses and dream of what might have been . . .

It is also perhaps the reason that Michelangelo and Leonardo da Vinci started to dress their boyfriends up in girls' clothes and paint them. There are no reports from the time of any boys, even the VERY sissy

ones, sitting around with gunge on their heads.

Men throughout Italy during this period made hilarious fun of the whole process and then, having done that, proceeded to show a marked preference for the mad women with blonde hair and rouged bazongas.

In 1589, Cesare Vecellio reported gleefully

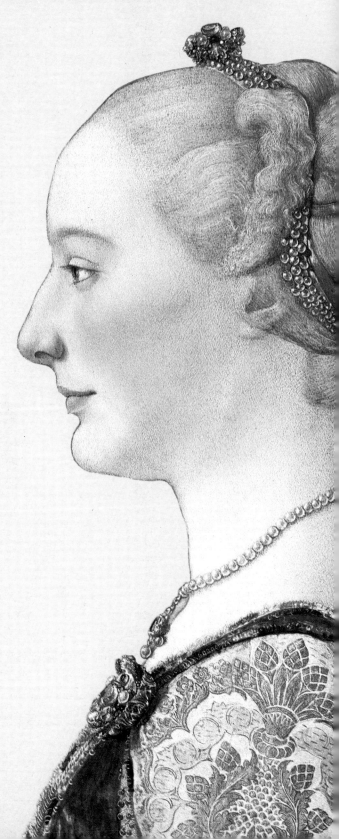

on a new way of acquiring the rare fair head. The houses of Venice were usually crowned with a little out-house affair, where the women would sit in the broiling heat all day. According to Cesare, 'it is there that they strain every nerve to augment their charms ... during the hours when the sun darts its most vertical and scorching rays,

they repair to these boxes and condemn themselves to broil in them unattended.'

To make matters worse, in 1593 angry reports reached the Vatican from incensed monks in Paris complaining that even the nuns were wandering the streets with their hair powdered and frizzed into bouffant hair-dos.

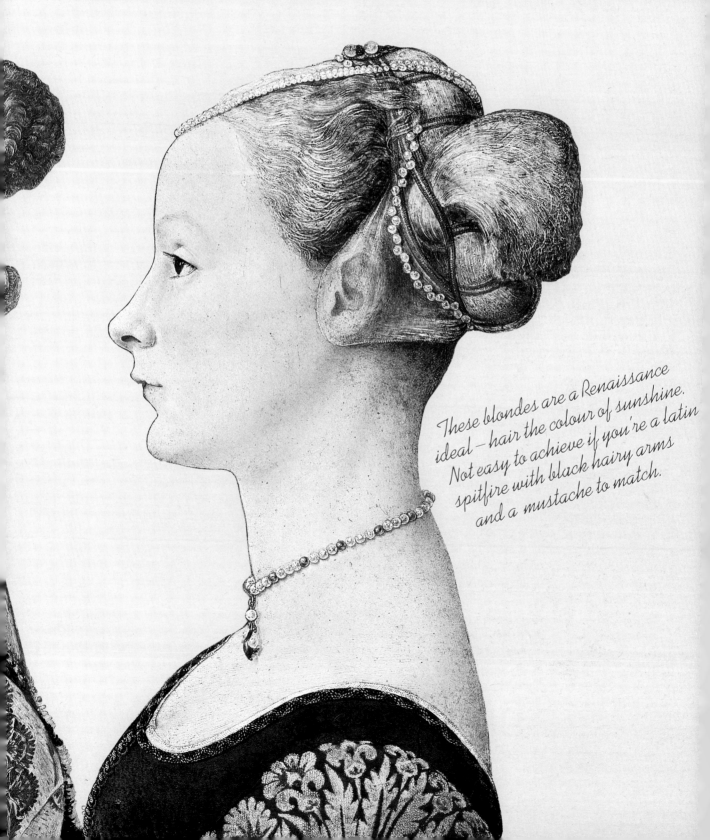

These blondes are a Renaissance ideal – hair the colour of sunshine. Not easy to achieve if you're a latin spitfire with black hairy arms and a mustache to match.

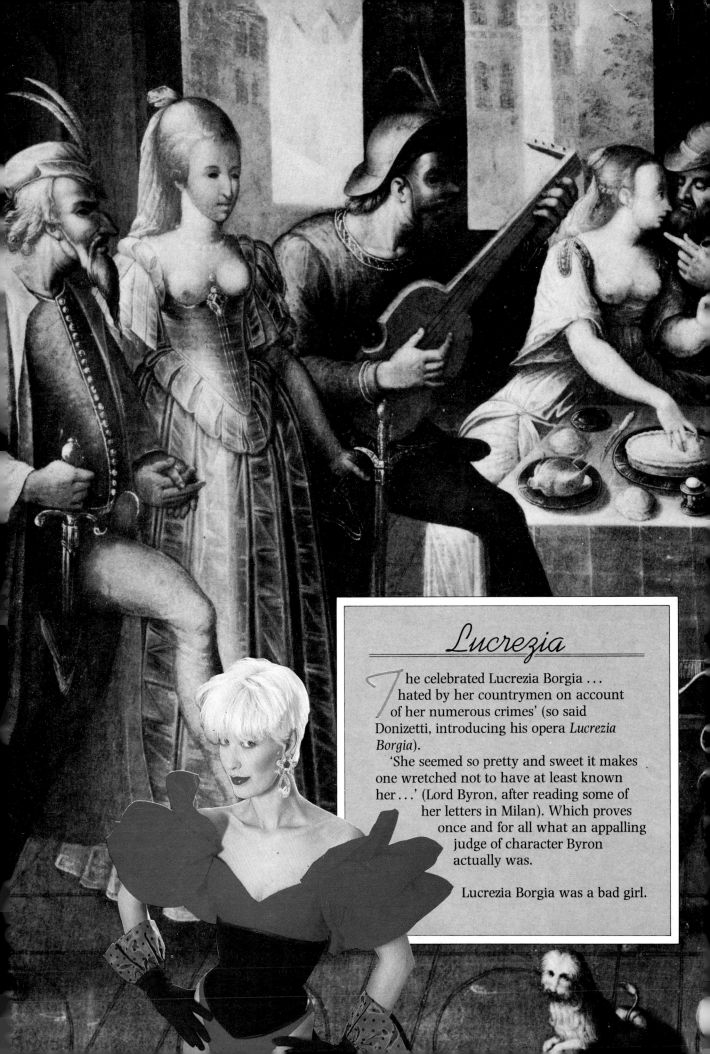

Lucrezia

The celebrated Lucrezia Borgia ... hated by her countrymen on account of her numerous crimes' (so said Donizetti, introducing his opera *Lucrezia Borgia*).

'She seemed so pretty and sweet it makes one wretched not to have at least known her ...' (Lord Byron, after reading some of her letters in Milan). Which proves once and for all what an appalling judge of character Byron actually was.

Lucrezia Borgia was a bad girl.

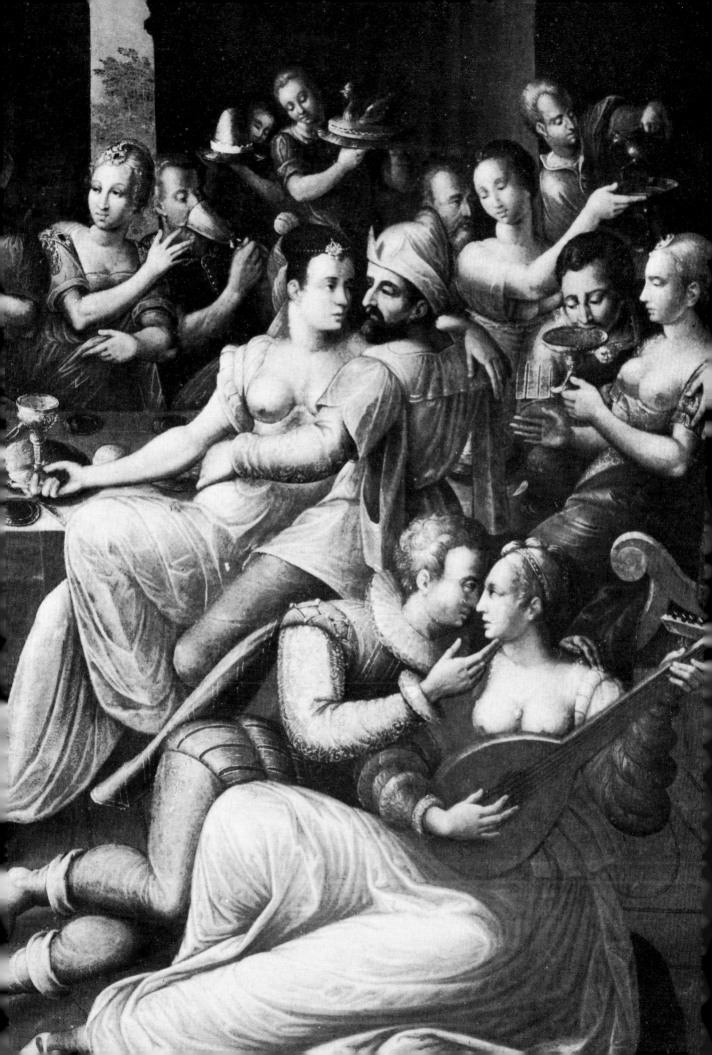

So naughty in fact that her family name has now come to represent everything that was corrupt and dangerous about the Italian Renaissance.

Her father, Pope Alexander VI, was commonly regarded as the wickedest of all the Popes, and Lucrezia herself as the most shameless hussy of her time. Reputedly she was not only giving one to her husbands, who dropped like flies but also having it off with both her father and her brothers. It was even rumoured that she had a child by her father.

Lucrezia and her best friend, Giulia Bella Farnese, were both notoriously blonde, and spent astonishing amounts of time fiddling with their hair – it was such a PERFORMANCE that one unknown poet of the day recorded their activities:

> What shall I say of the colour of their hair?
> That each one wants it long and blonde and beautiful
> But for this one must sit in the sun.
> What does it matter?
> Everything for this.
> They pay scant attention to their household
> and pass three hours looking at themselves.
> Drying themselves and curling themselves...

All this activity of course paid off. Lucrezia married several times. Men were attracted to her like moths to a flame, even though marriage to her was normally a very shortlived and dangerous affair which probably made it even more attractive.

After a number of false starts, Lucrezia's first marriage, decreed by Alexander, was to Giovanni Sforza in 1493. She was only thirteen at the time. In order to make her skin seem even whiter than usual Lucrezia, wearing white satin, had her train carried by a small black slave girl.

It appears that the Pope was rather dissatisfied with his son-in-law and decided to get Lucrezia out of the marriage almost immediately. He signed writs of divorce against Sforza, on the grounds of non-consummation because Sforza couldn't get it up.

Sforza was then faced with the sort of divorce case which would keep us all going for months if it were to happen now. He was faced with several choices, each one worse than the other, to prove that his wanger was in working order and always had been.

In the presence of witnesses agreeable to both of them, he could have Lucrezia brought to a neutral place and then demonstrate his technique upon her in front of them. If he didn't wish to subject Lucrezia to this humiliating experience, he could prove his virility on certain women in Milan approved by the court.

Sforza rather feebly claimed that he had 'known' Lucrezia a number of times and that the Pope was only doing this because he wanted her for himself. The Pope was having none of this: he needed a statement in writing from Sforza saying the exact opposite so that he could declare Lucrezia a virgin and get her another husband.

It is here that the story hots up even more. During the divorce proceedings, Lucrezia went to live in a convent with her ladies-in-waiting. Messages were brought by a handsome youth, Perotto, the Pope's chamberlain. He vanished and he was found six days later drowned in the Tiber. Lucrezia's lady-in-waiting, Penthesilea, was also found dead from drowning.

It appears from complaints from the Prioress that Lucrezia had introduced an unwelcome note of worldliness to her convent. There were rumours that she had got pregnant by Perotto. She was certainly pregnant by someone.

Penthesilea was the lady-in-waiting who had dressed Lucrezia during the sixth month of her pregnancy so that she could appear in court to hear herself described as 'virgo intacta'.

Seven months after the eventual dissolution of the marriage to Sforza, our virgin was due to marry again – this time to Alfonso, Duke of Biscaglia. Upon seeing the young man, Lucrezia apparently was hit by a thunderbolt of love at first sight. Upon spotting the blonde temptress, Alfonso obviously felt the same way. Gian Lucido Cattanei wrote soon afterwards, 'The daughter of the Pope appears most pleased

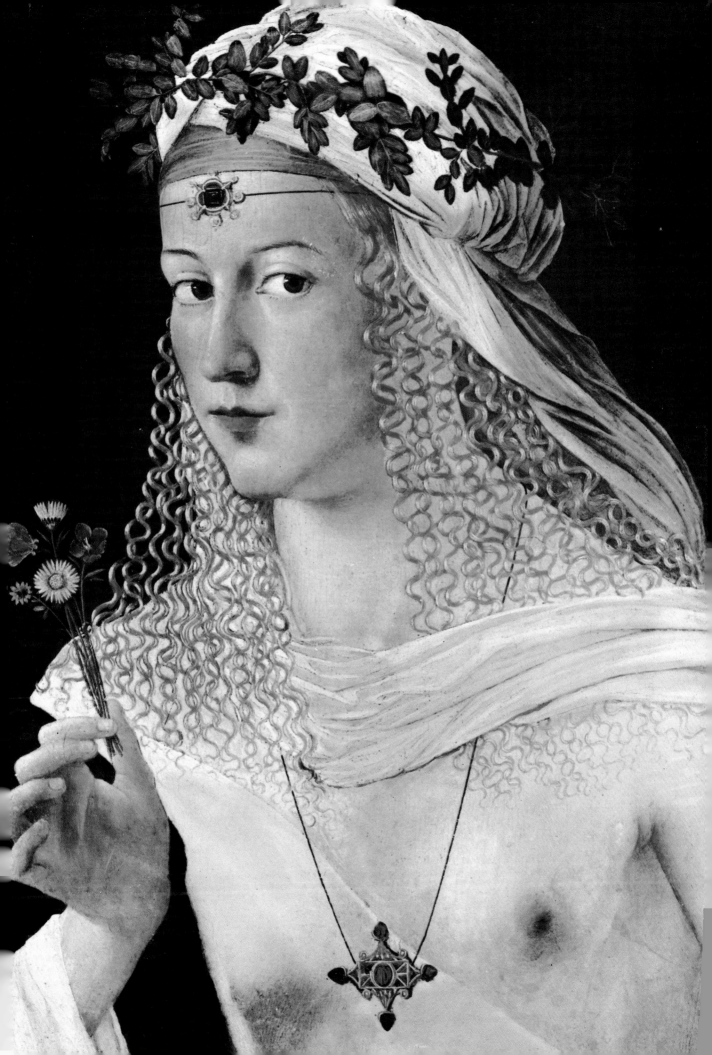

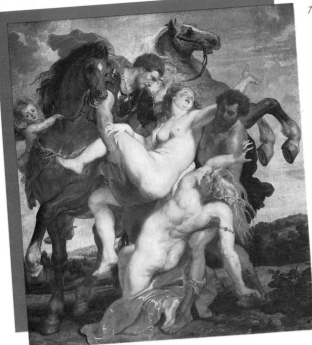

with Don Alfonso', and Burchard notes that the marriage was consummated on the first night (sez who?).

Not that all this blissful activity lasted. The next year, Alfonso was twice set upon by assassins and eventually strangled. It was rumoured that Lucrezia's brother Cesare was behind the murder.

Cesare sounds a pretty dodgy bloke anyway. Striding about in his wimple throwing parties of the worst possible taste all reported on by Burchard, who seems to have been Rome's equivalent of Jennifer's Diary.

He wrote of one party attended by fifty courtesans, who danced with the servants then took all their clothes off and picked chestnuts up off the floors, crawling naked on their hands and knees. Finally prizes were given to the men who were most successful with the prostitutes, the whole affair being watched by Cesare, the Pope and Lucrezia.

Burchard's diary places Lucrezia at another of these events, but this time the bodging was being performed by two mares and four stallions while the Pope and Lucrezia watched from the window above the gates of the Palace.

Lucrezia's journey into Ferrara from Rome for her next marriage was a grand affair like a latter-day starlet's entrance into

an epic film. Certainly she had enough luggage with her for at least fourteen other people. She had not particularly wanted to get married again, commenting in something of an understatement to her father, 'My husbands have been very unlucky.' But the man chosen to be her third husband was Alfonso d'Este, Duke of Ferrara, and this was to be her first meeting with him.

The journey to Ferrara was much the same as today's Royalty walkabouts, with Lucrezia making lots of small talk with people she didn't know from Adam in freezing cold weather and smiling all the time. This not only increased her fatigue from the journey but also added to her total panic over how she was going to look the first time she met the new flavour of the month.

When Alfonso came to collect her at two o'clock that afternoon she was dressed to kill. Knowing her temperament and reputation, he might have had a passing tremor that that meant literally.

She was wearing a camorra of gold cloth, with purple satin stripes. The gown had wide flowing sleeves lined entirely with ermine and an ermine lined cape made of gold-embroidered cloth-of-gold. So as not to appear as if she was trying too hard, Lucrezia kept her jewels to the minimum, wearing one of the two pearl caps which Alfonso had given her and a diamond-and-ruby necklace which was a gift from her new father-in-law. The whole assembly was naturally created to set off her long blonde hair to its best advantage.

Alfonso's procession consisted of seventy-five crossbow men in red-and-white livery, three captains and eighty trumpeters in purple-and-white stripes and cloth-of-gold, and the nobles and gentlemen of Ferrara. Seventy of these gentlemen were wearing large necklaces worth 500 ducats each (one ducat = £60), some wore necklaces worth 800–1200 ducats just to show who was who.

Alfonso's horse was wearing an interesting outfit made of purple velvet embossed in gold. The groom was wearing a slightly less colourful suit of grey velvet

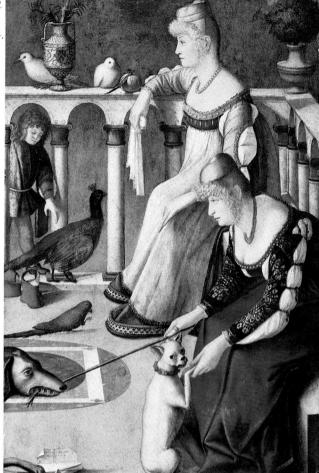

liberally covered in scales of beaten gold which the fashion pundits of the day estimated had cost at least 6,000 ducats and was obviously the sort of thing you spill your soup down the first time you wear it.

He was followed by eight squires in purple-and-gold outfits with red-and-purple striped tights à la Tony Curtis.

By comparison with all this showing-off, Lucrezia's men looked a little dowdy. Her twenty Spaniards were all dressed in black and only twelve of them had necklaces. After them came foreign ambassadors and bishops, walking two by two, and they were followed up the rear, in more ways than one, by six drummers, and two jesters who looked like they'd got their velvet outfits cheap at the sale at Bentalls.

But Lucrezia herself was a vision of gold, her spendid grey horse caparisoned in crimson and gold. Four of the professors from the University held a canopy of crimson satin over her golden glistening head and eight grooms fiddled with her horse constantly.

The only slight hitch in this wonderful ornate fabulous BLONDE event was when she finally rode over the bridge. She was saluted by blunderbusses which so upset her horse that he reared up and threw her on the road in a heap. Always ready to throw a shape, Lucrezia gave a merry laugh as she kicked the horse up the backside and mounted a little mule of her father's. This unpretentious act naturally captivated her audience.

Lucrezia emerged as a great leader of fashion from this moment. Women once again wore golden wigs to imitate her ravishing hair and carefully copied all the clothes she wore. She seems to have been happy hunting every day except on the days when she was 'washing her head' and planning dances and banquets for her husband. Despite this it does not seem that the marriage was a particularly tender one.

Before the marriage, Alfonso had frequented prostitutes 'because he felt he didn't know how to treat a woman of breeding'.

Nonetheless, upon her death – despite her terrible reputation for smutty business and poisonings – Lucrezia seemed deeply loved by her husband to whom she had borne seven children. He wrote to his nephew Frederico, 'I cannot write this without tears, knowing myself to be deprived of such a dear and sweet companion.' He then fainted at her funeral and had to be carried out.

The people who were generous about Lucrezia and grief-stricken by her death were however rapidly forgotten. The juicy stuff was much more worth repeating. Twenty years later the Neapolitan poet, Giovanni Pontano, getting back at Lucrezia's father for his ill-treatment of the House of Aragon, wrote of Lucrezia:

Here lies the tomb of a Lucrezia in name,
But a Thais in fact,
Daughter, wife and daughter-in-law of
Alexander VI.

The sixteenth century heralded the end of the free-for-all that allowed women to wear almost anything as long as they didn't look complete pilchards. The sixteenth century can be defined by its search for order, discipline and form in all things. For the first time dictates about how a woman should look in order to be conventionally beautiful, what she should wear and say, how she should behave were also decided.

The rules of beauty were numerous. Her hair should be a soft yellow, her forehead twice as broad as it was high, her skin transparent, her eyebrows dark and silky and most strongly marked where they tapered towards the nose and ears. The whites of her eyes were most odd, faintly touched with blue, her irises brown and not black, the lids delicately latticed with little red veins. The hollows of her face around the eye for example should have the same rosy glow as the cheeks. The flat part of the face should be paler than the hollows and, according to Firenzuolo's beauty book, with 'an edge of ruddiness as of a pomegranate'.

Elizabeth I

The love poems of Elizabethan England lavished attention on fair-haired women, mainly because the Queen, Elizabeth I, had strawberry-blonde hair of which she was inordinately proud:

> ... golden tresses loose (a joy to see)
> Which gentle wind about thy ears doth
> blow

> *Robert Tofre*

In return for such words a sensible system of payola was inaugurated. After a few stanzas the blonde would give the poet a small gift or token of her esteem. Next to being immortalized in paint there's nothing a blonde likes so much as being immortalized in print.

Elizabethan hair fashions included plucking the hairline to give it a heart-shaped effect and greater height – all in imitation of the Queen. She wasn't a great looker anyway.

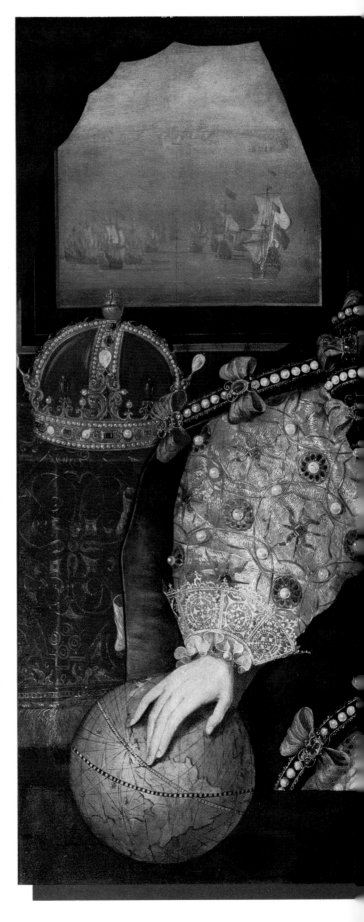

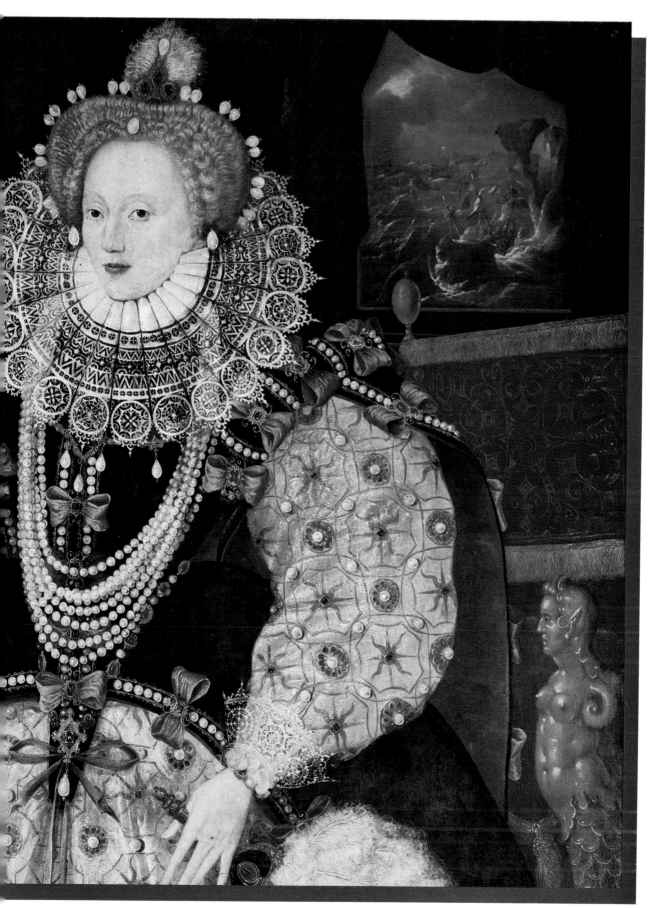

Elizabeth's skirts were vast to cover her numerous pairs of knickers — each with a pocket for a 2p in case she got lost and had to phone home.

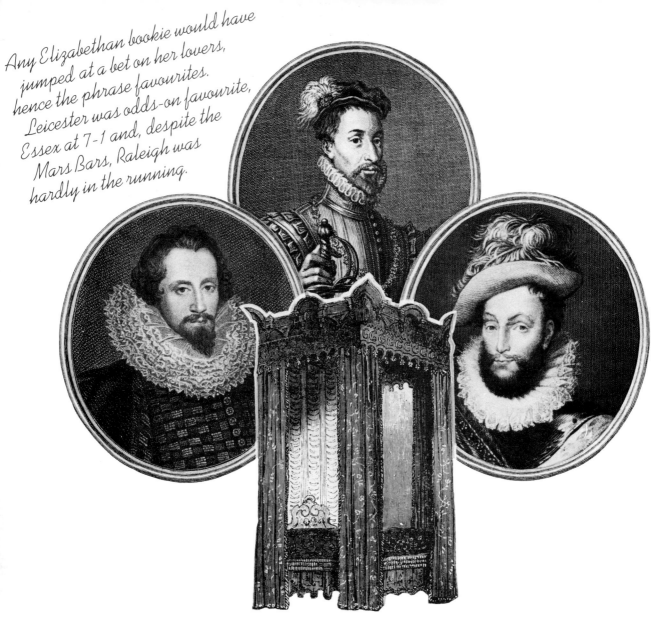

Any Elizabethan bookie would have jumped at a bet on her lovers, hence the phrase favourites. Leicester was odds-on favourite, Essex at 7-1 and, despite the Mars Bars, Raleigh was hardly in the running.

Elizabeth Tudor, like Madame de Pompadour, was an accomplished young lady able to speak five languages and do all manner of dances. She reigned over England for forty-four years and was one of its most popular monarchs. She was also a creature of contradictions. In her relations with women she frequently gave them a wallop if they displeased her. And she was famous for her 'favourites' – men who became close to her, got knighted, earled and duked, but never bodged.

Elizabeth was known as the 'Virgin Queen', nowadays something of a contradiction in terms in itself. Until her death in 1603, not only was she promoting geographical exploration and artistic adventure, she was also hanging on to her halfpenny like there was no tomorrow.

Elizabeth was proud to say, 'I am already married to a husband, which is the people of England.' So for thirty years the main gossip around the Court was, 'Does she or doesn't she?' It was undoubtedly in Elizabethan times that well-known phrases like 'I'll die if you don't let me', 'blue balls' and 'I'll only put a little bit in' first came into being, as the Queen's favourites hobbled from the bedroom praising her hair loudly and clutching their codpieces.

Like most of the great teases of our time, she adored being flattered more than she wanted the actual act. In a way this seems understandable. Why would she have wanted to share her crown with a husband, when instead she could have numerous devoted admirers panting around her like huskies. And very handsome huskies too.

She enjoyed the excitement and build-up of a mammoth crush with all of them without the nervewracking first night together, when you end up so nervous that you're doing raffia work on his bedside table at three in the morning.

Her longest affair was with Lord Robert Dudley. Rumours abounded that he had actually managed to make love to the Queen, but it does seem highly unlikely: even when she thought rather unromantically that she was dying of smallpox, she was still busily swearing on bibles that 'nothing improper had passed between them'. But lots of improper things happened to Dudley on the quiet so maybe that's how he managed to cope with lengthy sessions of romance where two hearts would beat as one, and Dudley would throb alone.

Yukie pukies what a thought.

As Queen, Elizabeth had to put up with the court gossips (the equivalent of the *Sun*), linking her name with all sorts of foreign princes and aristocrats, all of whom then turned out to look like Ethel Merman and worse. Philip II of Spain chased her, Archdukes Ferdinand and Charles of Habsburg pursued her, but after the usual system of sending a miniature of themselves, she sensibly decided they weren't the sort of boys anyone would want to kiss with their mouths open for fear of a bout of trench mouth.

Charles IX of France decided the best policy was to send someone else in his place to say the sweet nothings she so enjoyed, but he got sent back on the next ferry.

Most curious of her admirers was the smouldering homosexual, the Duke of Anjou, who was obviously willing to shut his eyes and think of England if it meant helping rule it. In the end he was spared having to practise his foreplay by the intervention of the Duke of Alençon, his younger brother, who almost succeeded in marrying Elizabeth – by now forty-nine and a rather grumpy blonde for a twenty-seven-year-old man. She managed to keep him hot to trot for almost eleven years, the rumours of marriage fuelled by the fact that the Duke was, as they say in Mandingo books, a man with 'mighty potent sap'. Unfortunately, sap or no sap he kicked the bucket at an early age and the Queen was said to be quite delighted.

Later in life she became really awful looking, the effects of lead in her foundation taking their toll. She loathed mirrors and could instantly fall out of love with her youthful favourites if they happened to catch her without her wig on in the morning.

She now spent a great deal on artificial aids, despite the fact that the Church moaned constantly about the use of wigs, saying they were 'the mark of the Devil'. A warrant signed by the Queen and dated 1602 orders payment for 'six heads of heare, twelve yards of heare curle, one hundred devizes made of heare'. The Queen is also supposed to have possessed a large collection of perukes, whatever a peruke is. Probably a wig for a perukie.

During her reign, with strawberry-blonde hair in vogue, various foul-smelling unguents were available for the daring boiler. One popular Elizabethan blonding agent consisted of 'the last water that is drawn off the honie being of a deepe red colour'. This transformed the hair to a golden glow. It also gave it the unique texture of a cabbage sprayed liberally with superglue.

When she died, Elizabeth said that she wished her epitaph to 'declare that a Queen, having reigned such a time, lived and died a virgin'.

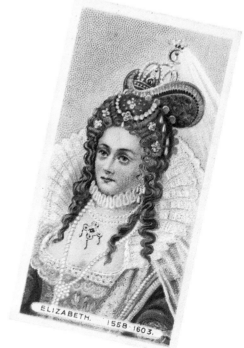

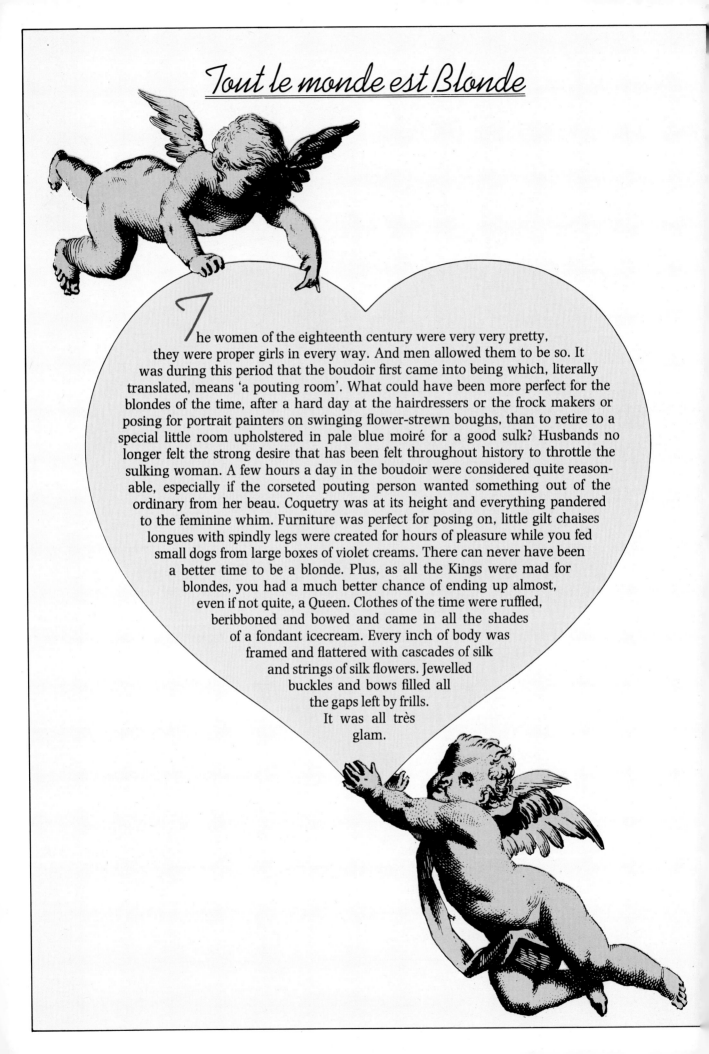

Tout le monde est Blonde

The women of the eighteenth century were very very pretty, they were proper girls in every way. And men allowed them to be so. It was during this period that the boudoir first came into being which, literally translated, means 'a pouting room'. What could have been more perfect for the blondes of the time, after a hard day at the hairdressers or the frock makers or posing for portrait painters on swinging flower-strewn boughs, than to retire to a special little room upholstered in pale blue moiré for a good sulk? Husbands no longer felt the strong desire that has been felt throughout history to throttle the sulking woman. A few hours a day in the boudoir were considered quite reasonable, especially if the corseted pouting person wanted something out of the ordinary from her beau. Coquetry was at its height and everything pandered to the feminine whim. Furniture was perfect for posing on, little gilt chaises longues with spindly legs were created for hours of pleasure while you fed small dogs from large boxes of violet creams. There can never have been a better time to be a blonde. Plus, as all the Kings were mad for blondes, you had a much better chance of ending up almost, even if not quite, a Queen. Clothes of the time were ruffled, beribboned and bowed and came in all the shades of a fondant icecream. Every inch of body was framed and flattered with cascades of silk and strings of silk flowers. Jewelled buckles and bows filled all the gaps left by frills. It was all très glam.

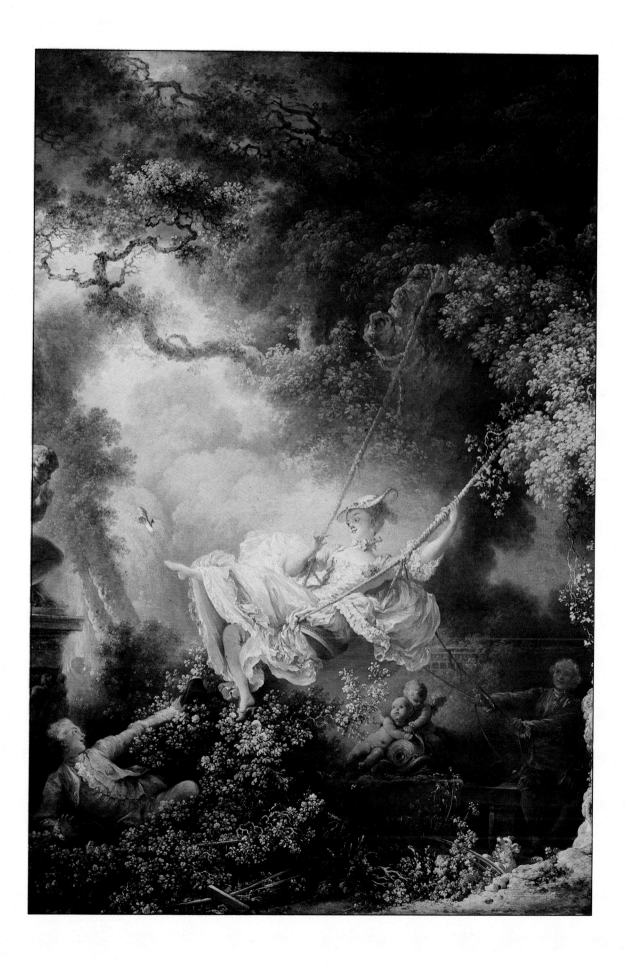

Beneath all the plump pink cupids firing their arrows across the ceilings of the great houses of France, it was however rumoured that while these ladies might have looked good enough to eat, you couldn't always be sure that they were. Had Fleet Street's telephoto brigade existed in the day of the French Court they would have died and thought they'd gone to heaven. No more nights spent freezing around Balmoral praying for a shot of the Princess Diana without her husky on. Ladies of the French Court thought nothing of the problem of not quite making it to the ladies' loo in time, despite all their frilly decoruming. Passers-by in the corridors of Versailles must have frequently come across heads covered with petticoats...

As one close friend of Madame de Pompadour remarked, 'Every corridor has a smell which reminds me of a special moment.'

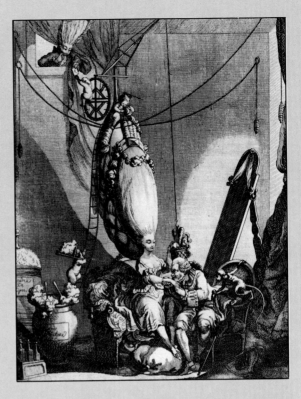

Elizabeth I had nothing on the eighteenth century in the hairpiece department. This was the true Great Age of the Wig, above all the powdered variety.

The fashion started in France, naturally, the French being a vain bunch.

Louis XIII started to wear a wig in 1624 – to cover up the fact that he'd gone bald at

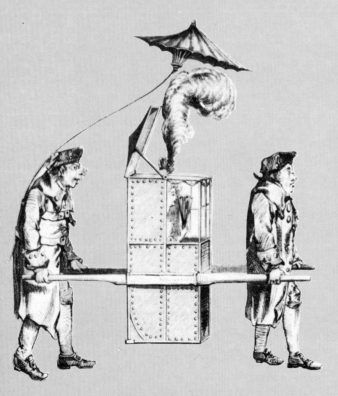

the age of twenty-four. The members of the King's court took up his lead and wigs rapidly became the mark of great wealth and leisure despite the fact that they made everyone look at least ninety.

Louis XIV was similarly self-conscious about the state of his head. Later on in life he allowed no one except his barber Binette to see him without his wig on. He wore a bed cap with a tassel on the end when he had his mistresses to stay the night. This was preferable to what would have been a dreadful sight, the King bollock-naked with his enormous white wig stuck into place cavorting around the four-poster. In the morning the curtains of his bed were always drawn and the King's wig was ceremoniously passed to him on a silver platter through a crack in the drapery.

Charles II of England introduced the wig to London dandies when he returned from an extremely pleasant period in exile. Being a sensible chap he hadn't exiled himself on any poxy island in the mid-Atlantic but had moved into Versailles until all was forgiven.

The wig was taken to London Society's bosom and literally hundreds of styles evolved. The eighteenth-century's equivalent of the New Romantics, a group of young men called the Macaroni Club, trolloped around town wearing vast toppling edifices which they spent hours perfuming, waxing and primping. They would frequently annoy staider members of society by whipping out their combs in public and fiddling with their giant toupees.

These wigs were astonishingly

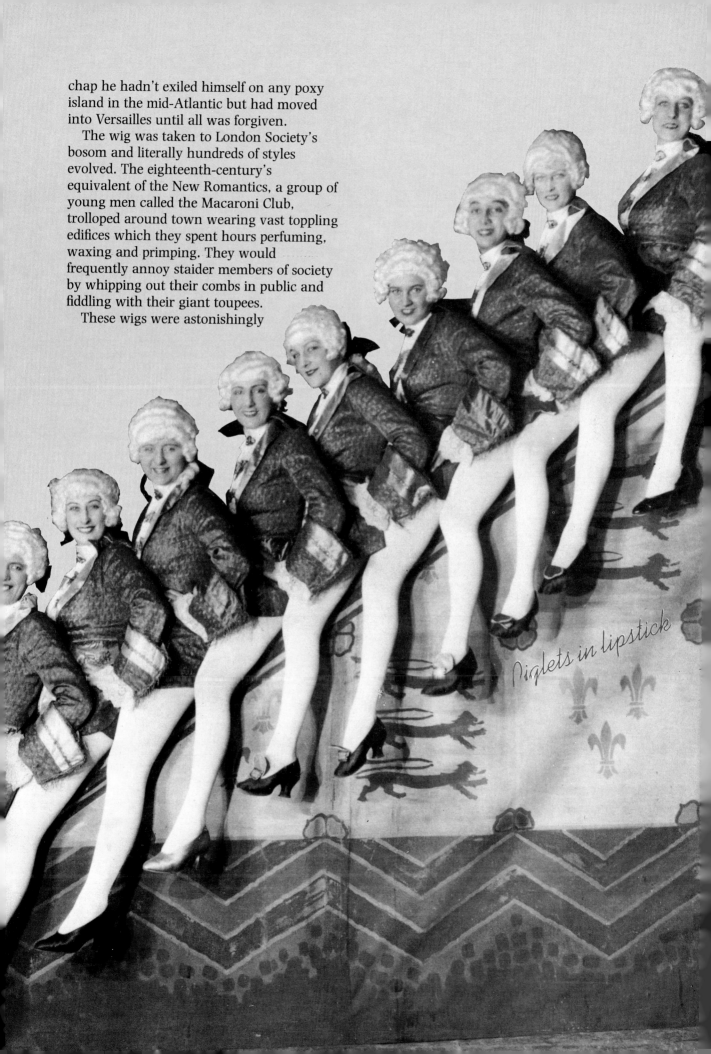

Piglets in lipstick

complicated constructions. In Sir John Vanbrugh's comedy, *The Relapse*, the wig-maker assures his client that the wig is so massive it will act as a hat and a cloak all at the same time. Meanwhile his client, aptly named Lord Foppington, notes that a really good wig should allow a woman to see nothing of a man but his eyes.

Women were not to be outdone in these absurdities. In France Madame de Lauzun wore an enormously high wig which had on the top a tableau consisting of what appeared to be a flock of ducks circumnavigating Cape Horn in bad weather, some rural scenes of shooting and the Hunt, and a mill with a miller's wife outside flirting with the local vicar while the miller was leading a donkey away. This extravaganza no doubt meant that Madame de Lauzun was never stuck for a conversation piece.

The newspapers on both sides of the Channel worked themselves into a lather of self-righteous annoyance over all this frivolity – rather like the reaction to Hot Pants in the early 1970s. The satirists had never had it so good.

In 'The Gentlemen's Magazine', hacks resorted to poetry:

To describe, in its dressing, the taste of the time,
(To answer your purpose, and fill up my rime),
Your choice must be made, for figure exemplar,
Of a Captain, a cit, a maccarroni, or a templar,
Let his figure be slender, and lounging, and slim,
Confoundedly formal, and akwardly trim,
Hang a hat on his head, let it squint fiercely down,
And be cut, slash'd, and scallop'd, and par'd to the crown,
Behind this strange head a quequ you must tye on,
Like a constable's bludgeon, or tail of a lion,
And before, when you try to embelish his hair,
Let your fingers be quick, and your powder be fair;
Be-friz it, and paste it, and cut it and curl it,
Now slope it in ranges, in rollers now furl it,
For the head of a fribble, or beau (without doubt),
Having nothing within, should have something without . . .

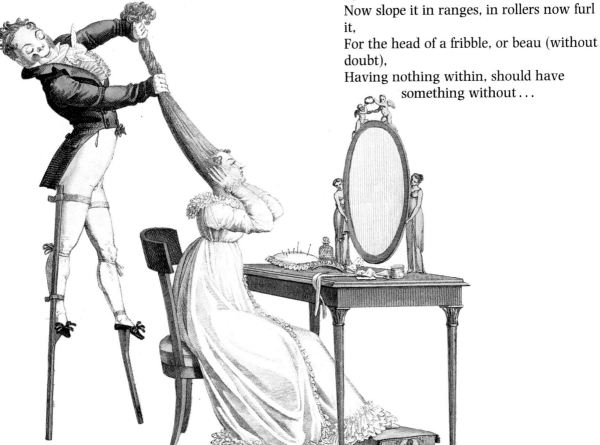

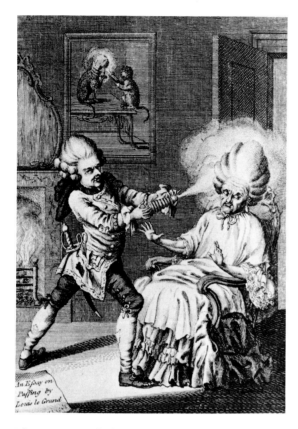

There was a slight hazard to all this glamour. Frequently mistaking the wigs for larders, animal life of all kinds found its way into them. Terrifying squashed creepies could be found on even the best scalps. The ivory and jewel-studded back scratchers popular at the time were in fact no such thing. They were used by wig-wearers who would weedle them under the edge of their wigs in an effort to scratch their bites and simultaneously dislodge any insects which had become embedded. Hairdressers rapidly dreamed up an answer to this problem. The theory was that if your pomade was sticky enough the insects would at least be stuck into position and were unlikely to roam to any more interesting regions of the wig-wearer's anatomy. The *pomatum* was made of beef marrow, smelled of Chappie. Powder was then blown through bellows at the wig: it rose in clouds all over the place, choking everyone involved. From then on, architects never designed a great house without a wig closet in which ladies and gentlemen could don their aprons and be powdered in peace.

Various substances had to be found for powdering wigs to the desired shade – lilac, pink, white or blonde. In the time of George II soldiers were issued initially with a pound of flour each week to put on their wigs, but at this shameful waste of baking ingredients the peasants rioted, so a search began for an alternative. One was a mixture of starch and plaster of Paris – which at least seems to have been guaranteed to keep it all in the air.

And so the unique relationship between the blonde and the hairdresser was born.

Marie Antoinette was devoted to her hairdresser, Larseneur – so much so that when his styles no longer pleased her she could not bear to get rid of him for fear of hurting his feelings. So he would come and dress her hair, and as soon as he left another hairdresser would arrive up the back stairs, unpick the whole lot, and start all over again.

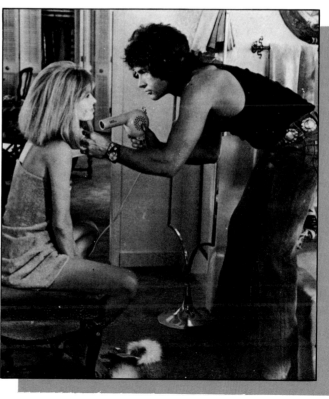

Madame de Fontanges

The leaders of fashion during this time were usually courtesans, who having captured the heart of a king or a nobleman were naturally felt to know their onions although kings notoriously have a taste for blondes of varying degrees of intelligence . . .

Madame de Fontanges was one of the many mistresses of the Sun King, Louis XIV, and she gave her name to a new hairstyle which she created accidentally while out hunting. Whether she was hunting bunnies or simply hunting the King remains to be seen but she returned with the King a besotted man. Fontanges was greatly romantic, physically exquisite and the possessor of all the intelligence of a broken milkbottle. The King was enchanted as he watched her riding recklessly through the countryside around Versailles on her little palomino pony in her pink riding habit, and set off in hot pursuit. Unfortunately as the King drew closer to her, she caught her flower-strewn hat on a low-slung branch, which knocked it to the ground. A born temptress, she jumped from her horse 'Dobbinette', and in full view of the King whipped up her dress, removed her lacy garter and tied her tumbling blonde curls up in that. The King promptly made her the Duchesse de Fontanges, and blonde cascades roughly tied up in lace soon appeared on every head, which the King thought delightful.

Madame de Fontanges couldn't have known the extremes to which the style would go. The cascade of blonde hair rose higher and higher and higher. It was stretched up on wire cones. In order that these masterpieces of scaffolding could endure, roofs, doorways and chandeliers had to be raised throughout Europe.

The style was forgotten in 1714 when Lady Sandwich arrived in the French Court wearing a small alluring hairstyle which naturally was immediately copied.

Blondes were probably relieved that they would no longer have to travel to parties kneeling in carriages with their heads poking out of the windows like Alsatians going to the seaside.

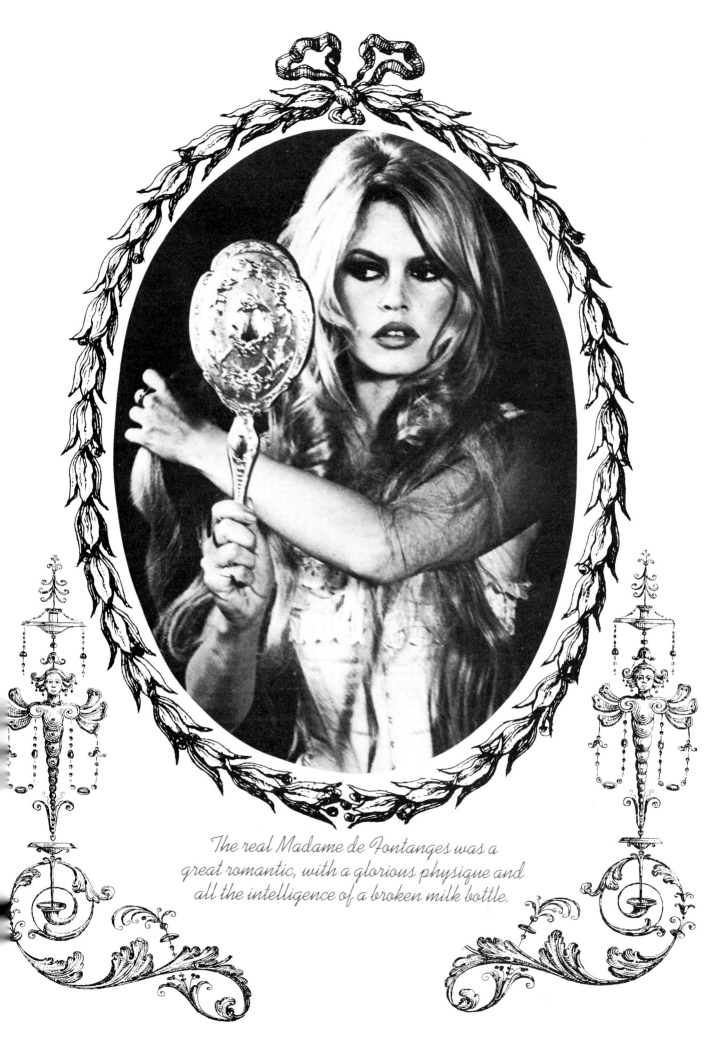

The real Madame de Fontanges was a
great romantic, with a glorious physique and
all the intelligence of a broken milk bottle.

Madame de Pompadour

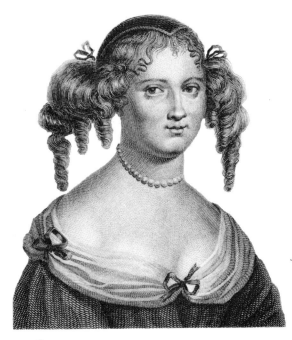

*T*he woman who perfectly epitomizes the eighteenth-century blonde is Madame de Pompadour. It should be mentioned that, far from being a staggering beauty, Pompadour bore a distressing resemblance to Dame Flora Robson had Dame Flora ever run in the Grand National.

Most biographers, wishing to gloss over the fact that she was a bit of a dog, say that painters found it hard to capture her prettiness because it depended upon her dazzle, gaiety and witty repartee as much as her bone structure. Bone structure? What bone structure you may ask, having perused the photographs. She appears to have worn a suet face-pack with two currants stuck in it for most of her portrait sessions.

The Marquis de Argenson loathed her with a ferocity not often seen among the wets hanging out at Versailles. He wrote his entire diary in the hope that his opinions of her would stick for posterity. He starts out mildly noting that she is 'tall and rather badly made' and then gets nastier and nastier. Finally he says that the King is tiring of her, that she spits blood, has black teeth and a scaly neck, and that her entire bosom is withering away.

Other diarists of the time say that the King was constantly falling more and more in love with her. That she spent entire afternoons on her swing with her legs in the air. Madame de Pompadour did most things with her legs in the air. The Marquis de Valcons wrote that 'with her grace, the lightness of her figure and the beauty of her hair, she resembles a nymph.' President Henault commented, 'she was one of the prettiest women I ever saw.' No mention of her scaly neck from those two devotees.

Madame de Pompadour was born, in the heart of Paris, Jeanne Antoinette Poisson. So she didn't do badly for a girl saddled with the name Jean Fish. She was the daughter of a woman of such beauty that virtually every biographer gives her a different father so wide is the possible selection.

At the age of nine Jeanne went to see a fortune teller who prophesied that she would one day rule over the heart of a king. From then on the entire family called her Reinette. One she had captured the King's heart she sent a special payment to the fortune teller.

Reinette was educated by two aunts who were nuns at a convent in Poissy. It must have been a fairly relaxed establishment because although she left it an adorable and accomplished creature she had no grasp at all of any aspect of the Catholic faith. But she could sing, dance and act, recite whole plays at once (sounds like a fate worse than death) and play the clavichord. She was a keen gardener who knew all about the new exotic flora and fauna that were being imported into France, she painted and engraved precious jewels and developed her exquisite taste in interior design, china and clothes.

So far from leaving the convent it seems she was an ideal mistress for any king – beautiful, talented and with an ability to spell rhododendron.

Her first meetings with the unsuspecting King were entirely manufactured by her. Although she was still officially married and

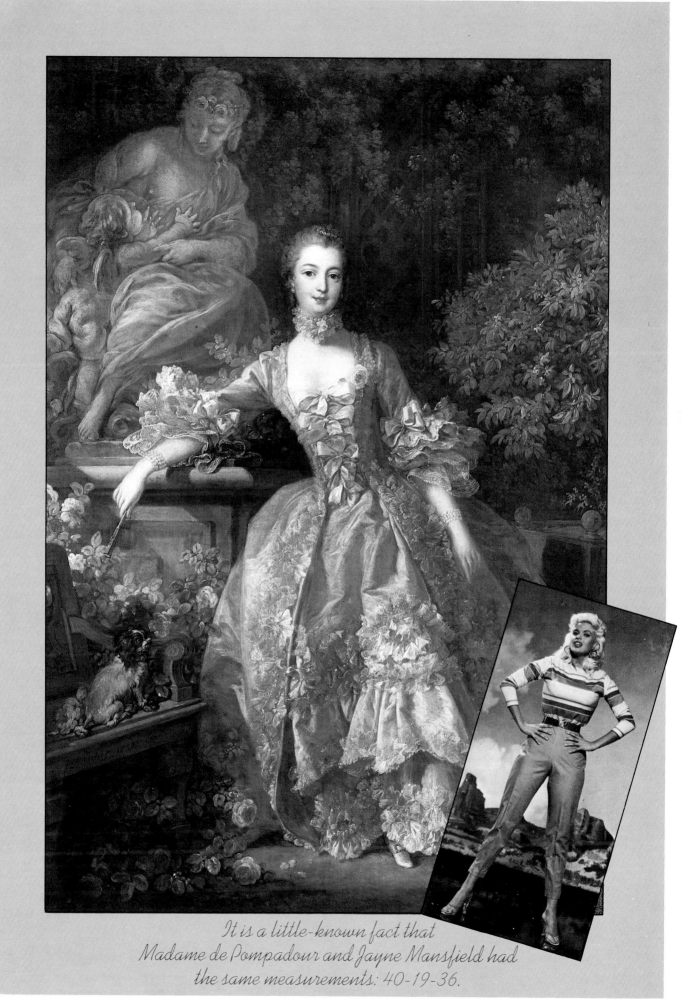

It is a little-known fact that Madame de Pompadour and Jayne Mansfield had the same measurements: 40-19-36.

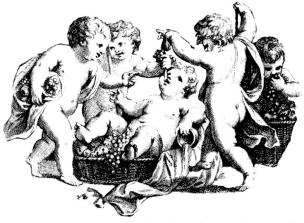

called Madame d'Etioles, she made sure that
their paths crossed constantly. While he was
out hunting she would recklessly ride past
him in her custom-built phaeton. If she was
wearing a blue frock she would drive a pale
pink carriage that looked as though it was
constructed from fondant icing. If she was
wearing sugar pink she would drive a pale
powder-blue carriage, and her white ponies
would run along with blue ribbons
streaming off them. Kings don't stand a
chance against these superior feminine
wiles.

For once, this King wasn't a man that
women loved simply because he was the
King. He was a French forerunner of Alain
Delon. He was tall, dark and very handsome
with a sultry brooding haughtiness which in
fact was a cover-up for his paralysing
shyness. Naturally all this smouldering like
a Gitane advert sent shivers of longing up
the spines of the ladies at the French Court.

Once the King became interested in
Madame de Pompadour, he was far too shy
to speak to her. In the end he decided to
send her a present. It wasn't very romantic
but it was a start: the King sent Pompadour
a fat grouse he'd shot that day.

He wasn't, unfortunately, the only person
who noticed her. His mistress Madame de
Chateauroux was getting rather wary. One
afternoon the two of them were enjoying a
quiet tea with the elderly Duchesse de
Chevreuse, who had known and adored
Madame d'Etioles since she was a small girl.
As soon as the conversation looked like
turning to the d'Etioles' many charms,
Madame de Chateauroux ground her heel as
hard as possible into the Duchesse's foot
rendering her temporarily speechless due to
severe lockjaw. Having nearly fainted clean
away the Duchesse had to go home to rest
her crushed foot in Epsom salts.

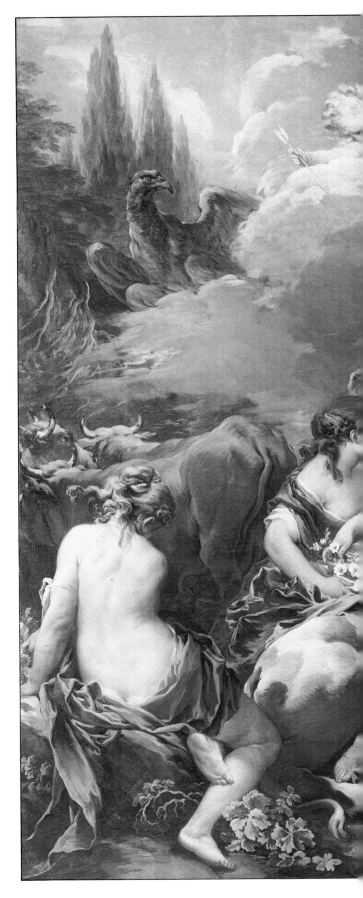

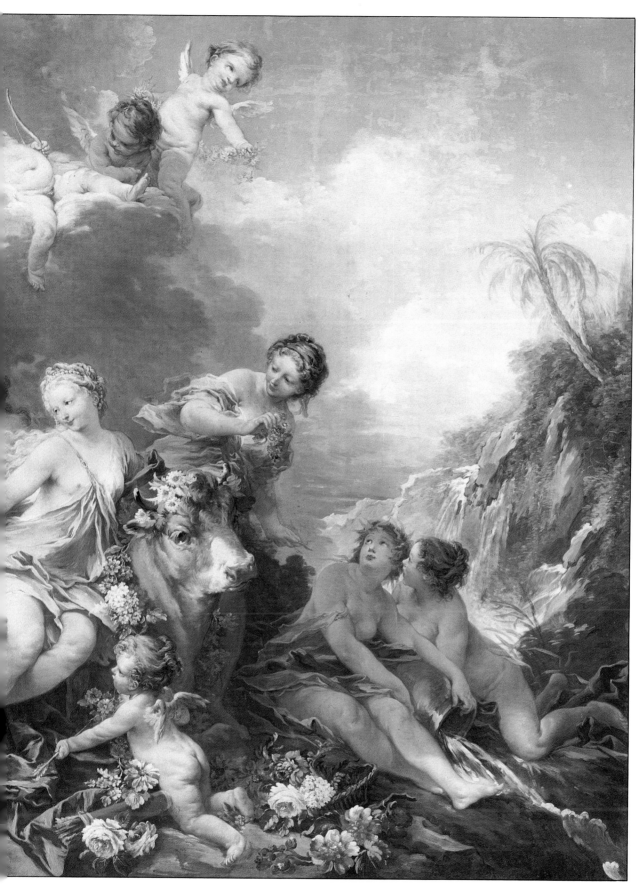

Versailles was Bunk-up Central.

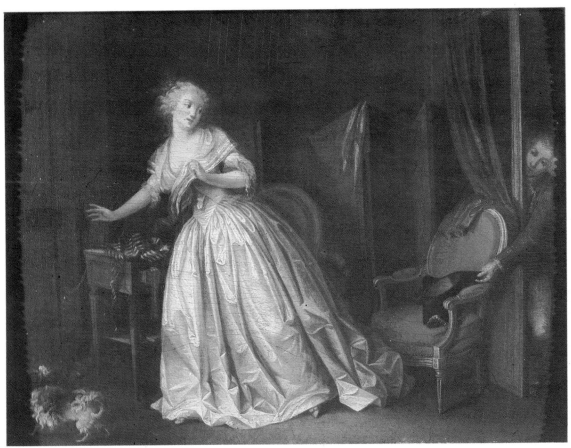

Scandals abounded at the French court, but bedrooms had more than one exit. Here, a girlfriend of Madame de Pompadour hears the local vicar approaching, singing 'Abide with Me', and sends her lover on his way pronto.

The next morning the contrite Madame arrived at the Duchesses's home to apologize. Her excuse, 'You know they talk of giving that little d'Etioles to the King...'

Probably by way of retribution for her foot-breaking activities, Madame de Chateauroux then died suddenly and the whole of Paris was agog at who would replace her as the King's true love.

Finally, after a great deal of tactics, Pompadour found herself at the ball of the Clipped Yew Trees. She was flimsily but appropriately clad as Diana the Huntress and she finally got her quarry. The King, convinced it was him that was the pursuer, unmasked himself to her next to a bush in the garden. As the fairy lights twinkled down on them the King arranged to meet her the following Sunday.

The King was enamoured with her for many reasons, which compensated for her pudgy face. She was funny and totally unscrupulous. She would entertain him as no other woman had done in the past. Pompadour had the blonde's natural interest in the seamier side of life. She got hold of the Parisian police reports each month and read the King the dirty bits; she also stole letters belonging to the more pompous members of the Court and read them aloud. In between all the sleaze she also did little dances and sang to him. The King had never experienced anything like it, certainly not with his wife who was a terrible bore and ugly as well.

But despite her great interest in other people's sexual activities, Madame de Pompadour didn't actually want to do it herself. The sexual side of their relationship didn't run smoothly, her velvety hand did not want to clasp the King's iron manhood at all. She began to be worried that she would lose his love if she didn't give him more attention in the bedroom. His demands became so incessant that Pompadour resorted to health foods to rekindle her fires.

She embarked on a diet consisting solely of vanilla, truffles and celery sticks. Not surprisingly after a week she was violently sick. Any rough motion of the bed made her even worse, defeating the whole object of the diet. The diets and aphrodisiacs finally bit the dust after a girlfriend of hers came to visit her and chucked all her truffles onto the fire. Pompadour threw herself onto the bed shrieking that she was not to be treated like a wayward child and never ate truffles again.

As the King's mistress, Madame de Pompadour had immense power over the King and his actions. Having a relation who's a mistress of royalty is useful to any family for precisely that reason. She soon had her friends move into their own rooms in the Palace and she embarked upon redecorating whole wings with her own

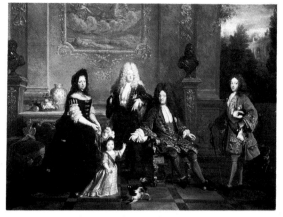

Louis XIV and his heirs – Louis XV is the one in the red satin knickerbockers.

taste. She then built her own wing to house the many treasures she'd collected together. The King never came home to an inactive household, the builders were always in.

Never before had a commoner, a member of the French Bourgeoisie, behaved the way she did. She made sure that there were no

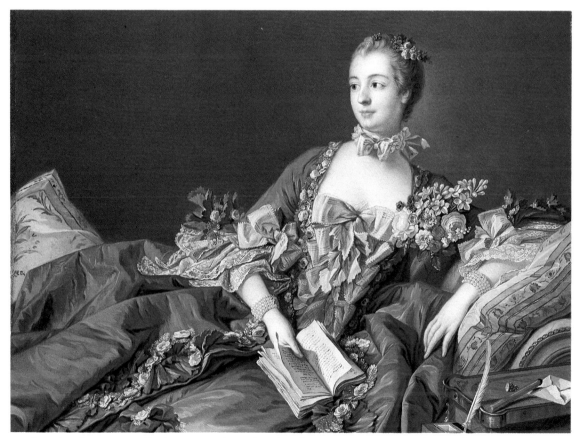

Not looking at all the sort of girl who does poo-poos in the palace corridors.

57

chairs in her bedroom except her own. Even Princes were forced to stand humbly before her. Only two men dared to do anything about this. The Prince de Conti sat smack on her bed and commented wryly, 'This is a good mattress,' and the Marquis de Souvre perched on the arm of her chair remarking, 'I didn't see anywhere else to sit.'

Madame de Pompadour was determined to retain her valuable position. She knew it was important for her to learn as much as she could about state affairs, and various aspects of politics. Despite her total lack of understanding of religion, she also decided that she should cultivate a more pious image. This she felt positive would cement her already strong position. Madame de Pompadour's conversion was one of the funniest in history . . .

The first thing she did, flinging herself back on her bed in a frilly pink peignoir, was declare loudly, 'I MADLY love the Holy Father', rather in the manner of Doris Day talking about Rock Hudson. She then went on a spending spree to equip herself for her new life as a devout Catholic. She purchased an illuminated prayer-book and crucifix from her favourite jeweller. She got her great chum Voltaire to translate the psalms for her, chatted endlessly to her friends about her 'state of grace' and 'the Christian life'. All in all she seems to have become the worst sort of born-again Christian. She charmed the nuns of St Cyr, where they called her the Vestal.

Gossip about Pompadour's new-found religious aura reached fever pitch when it was discovered that she had had the builders in again to block up the secret staircase linking the King's bedroom with her own. No one naturally liked to mention that there were still several others to exactly the same place. It was the pious thought that counted.

Pompadour then contemplated her next big step in the religious life. She was going to give up wearing rouge. But finally, after hours of contemplation, she decided that that was going too far for even the most devout girl on earth.

What Pompadour wanted to do more than anything was to be allowed to take her communion in public. She called in a Jesuit priest named Père de Sacy who gently told her that a woman whose hairdresser was known to be earning more than a quarter of a million dollars annually and who lived openly with the King could hardly expect the Church to regard her as the ideal advert for them. She indignantly explained that her relationship with the King was a chaste one and even told him of the blocked-up staircase as extra proof. The Father patiently told her that all she could do to rectify matters in the eyes of the Church was to return to her husband at once.

Here Pompadour knew that she was on reasonably safe ground. Her husband was living in great comfort with his mistress and the one thing he wouldn't want was the return of a repentant rougeless religious Pompadour after all their years apart! She wrote to him immediately and he responded exactly as she knew he would do. This letter she showed triumphantly to the long-suffering priest, adding that the King would never consider her leaving Versailles as it would make his life not worth living.

Eventually she did find a priest lenient enough to allow her to take communion but even he insisted she did it in private . . .

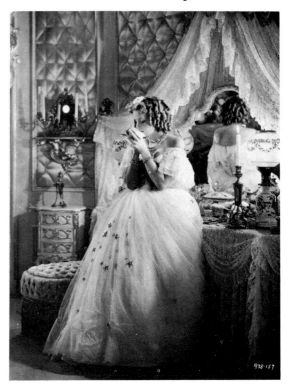

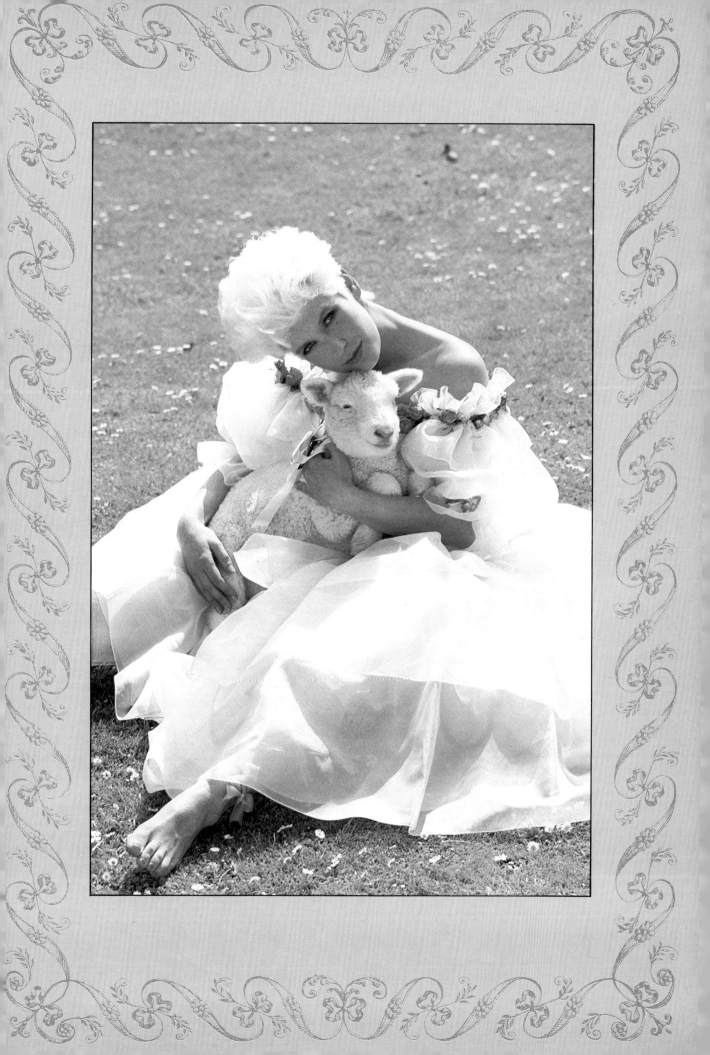

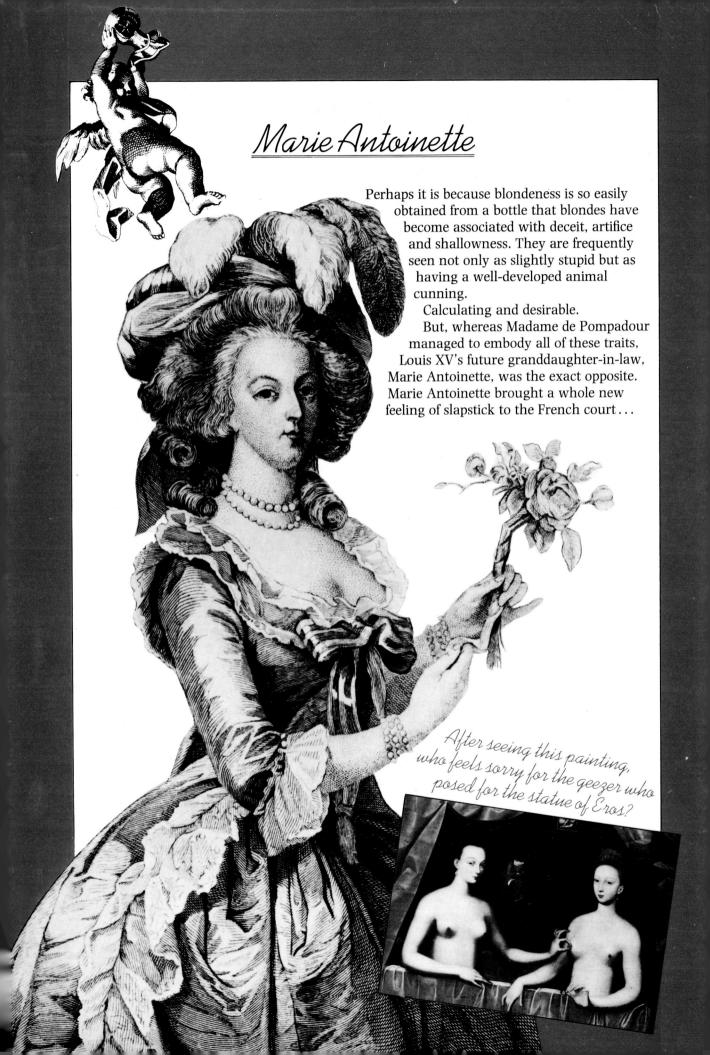

Marie Antoinette

Perhaps it is because blondeness is so easily obtained from a bottle that blondes have become associated with deceit, artifice and shallowness. They are frequently seen not only as slightly stupid but as having a well-developed animal cunning.

Calculating and desirable.

But, whereas Madame de Pompadour managed to embody all of these traits, Louis XV's future granddaughter-in-law, Marie Antoinette, was the exact opposite. Marie Antoinette brought a whole new feeling of slapstick to the French court...

After seeing this painting, who feels sorry for the geezer who posed for the statue of Eros?

Before becoming the Queen of France, Marie Antoinette, Archduchess of Austria, had a number of obstacles to get over. The first one was that she had two left feet and was entirely incapable of doing any of the fashionable dances of the time without either crippling her partner or resembling a country wench at the local hoe-down after one-too-many ciders. From 1768 onwards she was entrusted to one of the most famous dance teachers at the Paris Ballet, but to absolutely no avail. She learnt nothing, or almost nothing, despite the sweating efforts of her teacher to explain the glories of movement, which ended with him wretchedly chalking an X on her right foot as a clue to its whereabouts in times of need on the dance floor.

Two bits of self-improvement did go well. Firstly, she had terrible teeth, quite rotten and badly placed, but a French dentist summoned to Durfort on the Abbé Vermond's advice succeeded in clearing up her problems and by 1769 her teeth were pretty and in the right places rather than sticking out at right-angles as they had done before.

The second problem was her hair. It was the perfect ash-blonde colour, but sadly it grew from about an inch above her eyebrows giving Marie the somewhat neanderthal appearance that any blonde temptress could do without, especially with black buck teeth and two left feet...

Another Frenchman was sent to assist her with this problem and he invented a style which entranced the Viennese and which she later wore for her portrait by Ducreux, as Dauphine of France. The Count of Neny declared, 'It is simple and decent, but at the same time very flattering to the face', and he added, 'I am convinced that our young ladies who for some time have been wearing mountains of curls will abandon them forthwith and dress their hair like the Dauphine.'

It was now that the blonde and almost ravishing Marie Antoinette and her French hairdresser, Larseneur, began their friendship which she continued even after she no longer liked his styles. And quite right too since he'd given her a hairstyle fit for a crown.

The union between the Archduchess of Austria and the Dauphin of France was more than just any ordinary wedding. For two centuries the two countries had had endless wars and the Austrian menace had become a total obsession to the French. But by the time of Marie Antoinette, the Austrians and the French were united in a common fear of the expansionist policies of Prussia and England.

A pavilion was specially constructed for the meeting between Marie and the Dauphin on neutral territory and so as to make doubly sure of no rows it was also divided into two parts, one Austrian and one French. The French side was marked by two tetchy-looking greasers in striped tee-shirts and berets.

The French loved Marie on sight, as they appear to have managed to love anything associated with royalty. The Baroness of Oberkitch saw her for the first time that day and many years later wrote:

At that time, her Highness the Dauphine was tall and well made, although a little slim. She has changed but little since then; her face is still the same, long with regular features and aquiline nose although it has a Roman bridge; a high forehead [!] and lively blue eyes ... she had the Austrian lip.... Nothing can describe her dazzling complexion, literally milk and roses. Everything about her betokened greatness of her line and nobility of heart. She appealed to all...

Not quite all in fact, at this point. Louis XV presented to her the scowling young Dauphin, who had rigor mortis from terror at meeting his future wife in front of so many people. A cosy supper had been prepared later on for the royal party and Louis XV, feeling mischievous, invited his current mistress Madame du Barry to dine with them – which would have been regarded as a great insult to the young couple had Marie known at the time who

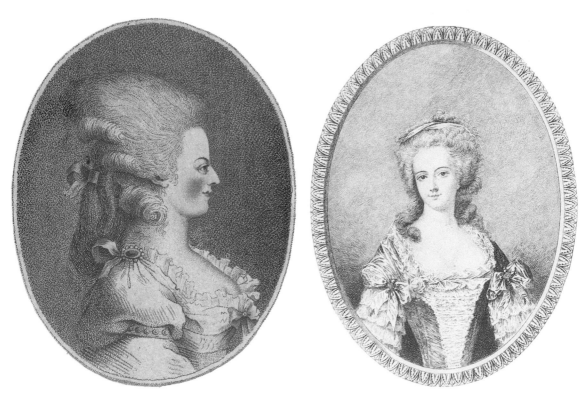

Marie Antoinette displaying the hairstyle that stopped her marriage being consummated for seven years.

Madame du Barry was. Luckily she did not, but once she discovered the insult later she always harboured a grudge against Madame du Barry.

That night her mind was on higher things. The King had a magnificent opulent casket of jewels placed in her bedroom which kept her occupied for some time trying on everything and jigging around. As a more personal gift she was presented with her own set of diamonds which was enough to put anyone in a good mood.

After the wedding ceremony at Notre Dame of Versailles, Louis XV signed the register with his clear hand, Louis Auguste wrote his name clearly and Marie Antoinette accidentally tripped up and made a huge blot with a smudge next to hers. Her reign of terror had begun ... But not that night. The newly-married couple, aged sixteen and fourteen years, went straight to bed and fell asleep. The marriage was not consummated for another seven years, which seems a trifle excessive even for them. He was probably sticking it in her ear.

When, in June 1773, the pair of them made their official entrance into Paris, the Duc de Brissac showed Marie the crowd that had gathered there to greet her. 'Madame, there before your eyes are two thousand people who love you.' The market women, according to an ancient custom, were then allowed to chat to the young couple and immediately gave them some advice regarded by all to be rather close to the bone regarding their marital problems which had been heard about throughout Paris months before.

Marie Antoinette appears to have made up for her husband's shortcomings by taking up other interests. She had a passion for cards and gambling and on one occasion played cards for thirty-six hours. After a few more of these marathon sessions her debts at the end of 1776 amounted to about a hundred million francs.

Not that Louis XVI minded. He attempted to make up for his fumbling as a husband and suitor by complying with every one of Marie Antoinette's whims. And if there was one thing she had in abundance, it was whims. The Queen was incapable of saying no to a jeweller's window whatever the state of her bank balance at the time.

In 1776, on an impulse, she bought herself a pair of earrings for £348,000. The King ended up paying for them on hire purchase for the next six years. Another shopping spree ended with her buying bracelets worth £162,000, which must have nearly given Louis a coronary.

It was probably because of the Queen's extravagant eye for beauty that Louis decided he'd better give her one to keep her out of the shops for a couple of hours every day, for in August 1776 the news spread through Paris that the marriage had finally been consummated. So delighted was the King at his achievement that he told Marie Antoinette, 'You like flowers? Well, I have a whole bouquet to give you,' and he gave her Le Petit Trianon, her country retreat. In his eyes, probably 'retreat' from the shops, with any luck.

In 1781 Marie Antoinette gave birth to her second child – a son – and the great celebrations commenced. After that began a long period of undeserved unpopularity and later hatred, which she met with thoroughly bad PR.

For Marie Antoinette, the situation was more serious than anyone realized. She had come to represent High Society and people now despised it. She embodied coquetry, extravagance and frivolity and whim at a time when the people of France were questioning all their values.

The Queen's wardrobe – said to contain 170 articles, and each year everything given away and new things bought at a reputed cost of £80,000 – her jewels and card playing were all seen as the proof and the epitome of the lifestyle which was now loathed.

At 12.15 on 16 October 1793 she was executed and the crowd shouted 'Long Live the Republic!'

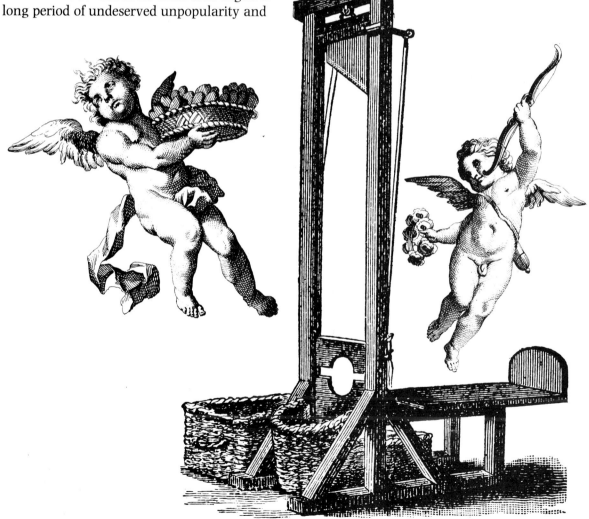

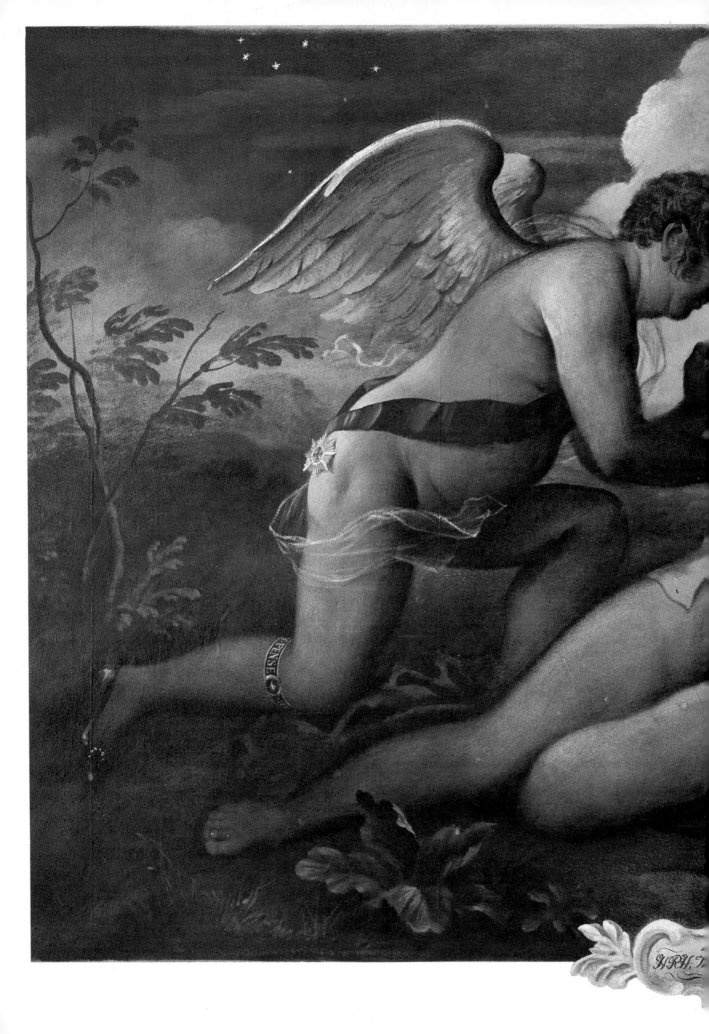

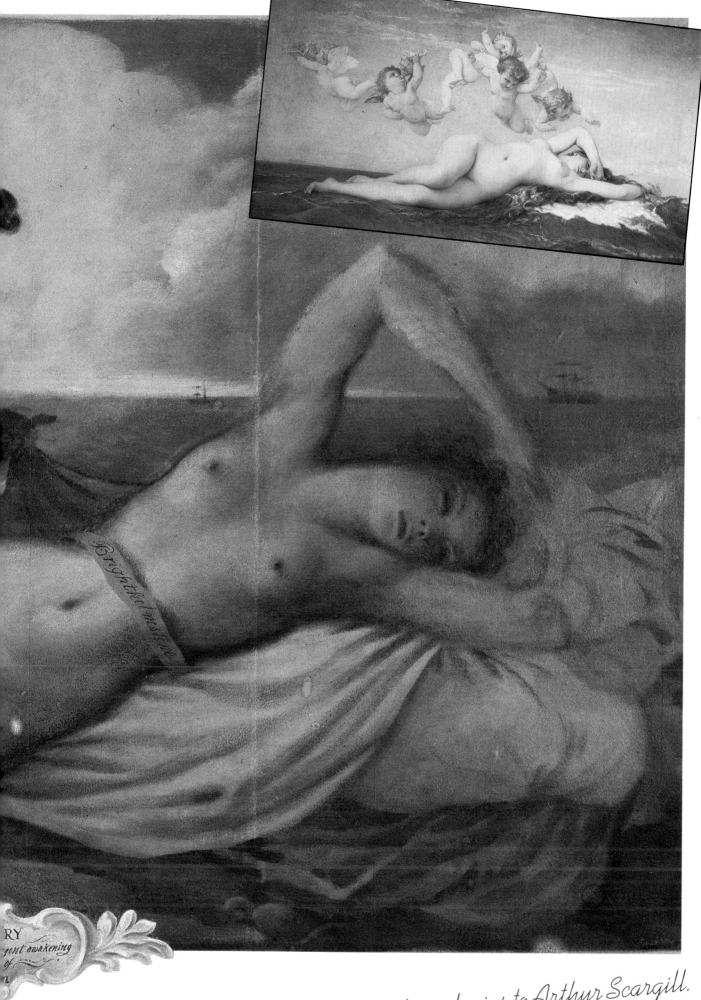

With apologies to Arthur Scargill.

The Repressed Blonde

Lo! as that youth's eyes burned at thine, so went
Thy spell through him, and left his straight neck bent
And round his heart one strangling golden hair.

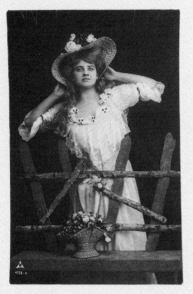

So the nineteenth-century poet Dante Gabriel Rossetti described Lilith, a legendary blonde whose beauty captivated and destroyed men. According to the average man-in-the-street at the time, most blondes were slightly evil goddesses likely to truss them up like oven-ready turkeys with yards of golden hair. The poor repressed Victorian man – tied to a brunette who spent entire afternoons reading Mrs Beaton's home maintenance book and writing in to agony columns about whether she should remove her gloves before shaking hands with a second cousin – spent hours contemplating all the things he felt sure that a blonde would do to him.

The German poet Goethe warned men against the special potency of blonde-haired women and their universal appeal:

Beware of her fair hair for she excels
All women in the magic of her locks;
And when she winds them round a young man's neck
She will not let him free again.

All of this anti-blonde propaganda naturally left men feeling mildly terrified of blonde temptresses. It was during the late 1850s that the first adverts became popular and this is where the blonde came into her own. Temptresses may be frowned on at coffee mornings but no one would say no to being one.

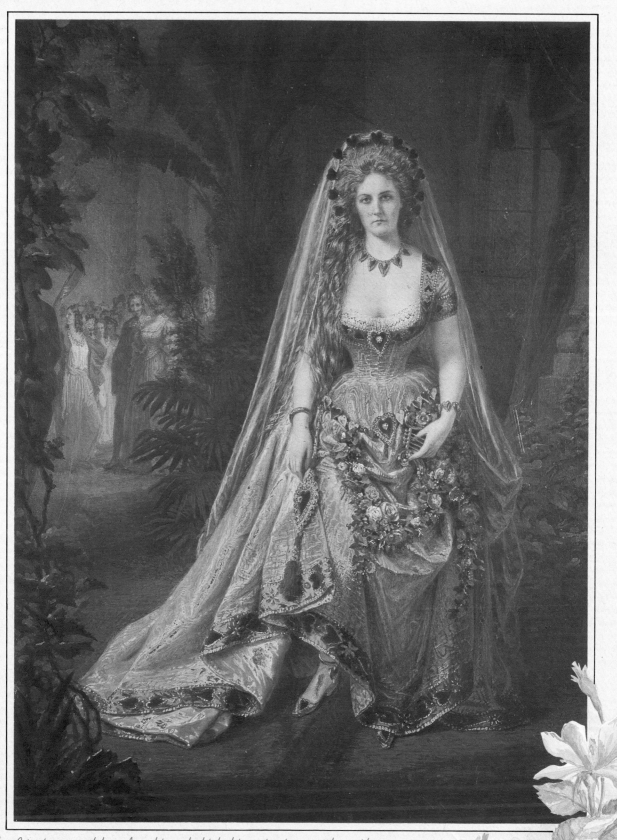

*The Victorian blonde often felt left out at social gatherings:
at balls like this she would end up
all alone, practising the language
of fans on a drunk aspidistra.*

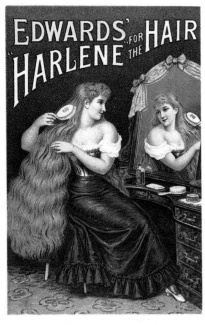

EDWARDS' HARLENE "FOR THE" HAIR

So adverts started to appear featuring all the charms of large-busted blondes wearing low-cut dresses with enormous bustles. As with everything else, the bigger the better appeared to be the nineteenth-century advertiser's motto. The first thing they did was extol the many virtues of the 'wave'. The reason that blondes were used to advertise this new hair torture was because their hair showed up the twin ridges considerably better, and with printing at the stage it was then this was of great importance. Perming and waving had become very popular and therefore big business. For those unfortunate enough to have straight hair, the effect was created by what appears to have been a rather fanciful waffle-maker which produced two or three ridges of hair on each side of the head. This looked like a small relief map of the Rockies on some young ladies but was still much sought-after, and the machine claimed to do the trick in only three minutes.

Even during the lean years for blondes, back in the 1850s, they were used to advertise awful things that needed glamour, something which still goes on today.

In the meantime those without blonde hair were striving to acquire it in as discreet a way as possible. Discretion was the name of the game when it came to dyeing. Golden and silver powders were on sale and also foreign blonde hair could be bought. It was imported from Belgium, France and Germany. German hair, the fairest and heaviest of all, weighed between $\frac{3}{4}$ and $1\frac{1}{2}$ lbs in weight and was naturally the most desirable for wig making.

After going to all this trouble to acquire the false hair, Victorian women also wired large white lilies to their ears and the napes of their necks to give them the appearance of walking funeral parlours.

Some racier types were actually dyeing their own hair with a potent bestseller alluringly called 'Golden Hair Fluid'. Despite the fact that because of its high content of ammonia and peroxide Golden Hair Fluid smelled of monkey's pee-pee, it was being liberally applied to scalps of the fashion-conscious across London. It was also priced according to where it was being sold which led to some interesting discrepancies. In the West End where it was sold in chic hairdressing salons (probably under the counter in a brown paper wrapper) it was two shillings, but in poor areas like Hackney, Stepney and Islington it sold for less than a penny in the grocers.

By the 1890s some heads looked unlikely ever to recover from the damage the peroxide had done, drying and breaking off in handfuls. Hair snapped at the sight of a hairbrush.

But good words were being said for blondes. A German gynaecologist writing in 1899 decided once and for all what he felt the reasons were for the blonde's appeal. Of course, he said, it suddenly dawning on him one summer afternoon as he searched for edelweiss in the Austrian alps – men love blondes because their fair hair harmonizes so well with the soft outlines of a woman's body. He hastened to add that while he felt that a woman's hair in her armpits should be also fair, her pubic hair should be dark to emphasize the width of her pelvis and the angles to her thighs.

Despite this seal of approval, of course dyeing had its critics.

One doctor rather unromantically described all blonde hair as simply an excess of sulphur and a deficiency of carbon. Another medical man from Bristol did his own bit of market research and came up with these results: out of 735 women in Bristol, only 33% of blondes were married. In the brunette group, 79% had achieved

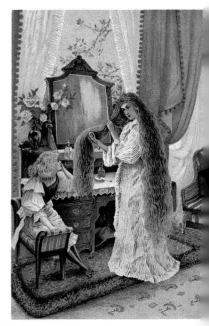

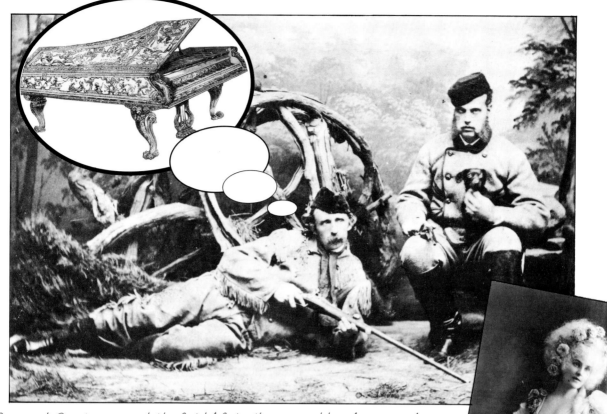

General Custer, one of the Wild West's many blondes, wondering whether to shoot the Russian Grand Duke Alexis' pet doggie Growlsky before he eats any more beans. Alexis, over to shoot buffalo, thinks of a pretty piano he met, and Growlsky sensibly dreams of the actress Madge Lessing.

this state of heavenly bliss.

Isabel Mallow went even further. She was a journalist of repute. She was also to hair dyeing what Mrs Whitehouse is to BBC2's epics about the Fall of the Roman Empire. During the 1890s she wrote regularly in *Women's Home Journal* on the topic of hair care. She sternly admonished her devoted readers:

> It goes without saying that a well-bred woman does not dye her hair. If in some moment of, I was going to say, temporary insanity, she should be induced to do so, although it would be mortifying and she would have to permit herself to look like a striped zebra for a short time, still it would be wisest to face the situation and allow the hair to grow back to its natural colour.

Dying one's hair blonde and having one's kiss curls in the wrong position were not the only things to make Mrs Mallow's hackles rise like an inflamed pekinese's ... 'Who of us have not grieved,' she wrote touchingly in her column, 'at seeing a friend, intelligent and pretty, make herself look stupid and ugly by an over-heavy fringe, frizzed like wool and made to come so far down on the forehead that there is doubt as to her ever having had one?' No doubt a million Victorian hearts nodded in unison at the thought of all their friends blonded and frizzed looking like sheep.

But Victorian women had a tendency to follow such insecure fashion trends. Painting the veins across one's bosom frequently went awry due to the lack of light in the bedroom. Ladies would emerge for a night on the town with a map of the Northern Line painted across their chests, their bosoms looking like stilton cheese with large blue veins running hither and thither – obviously racing up to the point where they could meet with the Victorian Ladies' Fringe.

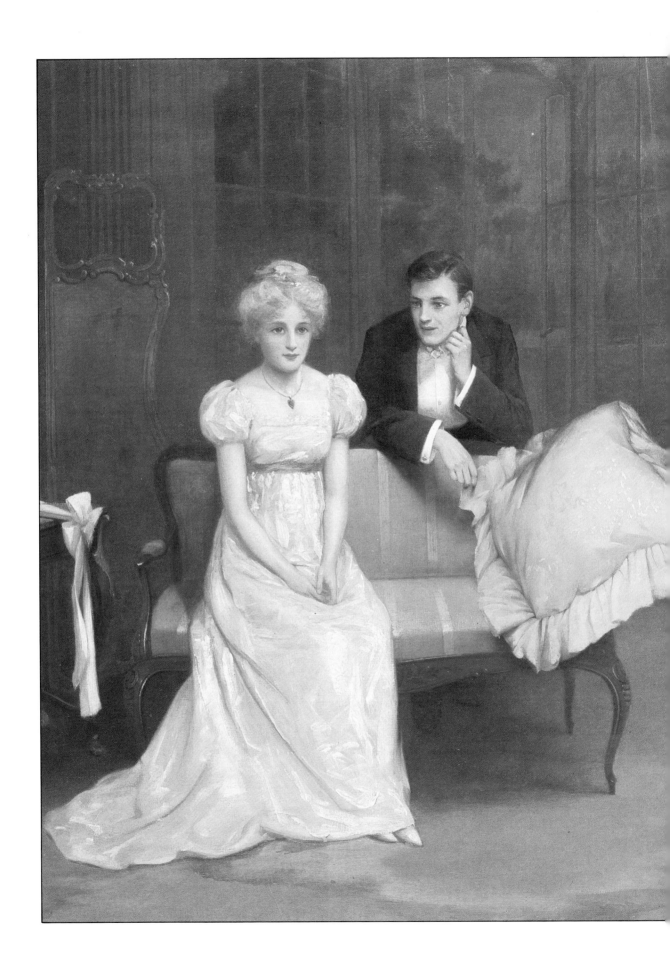

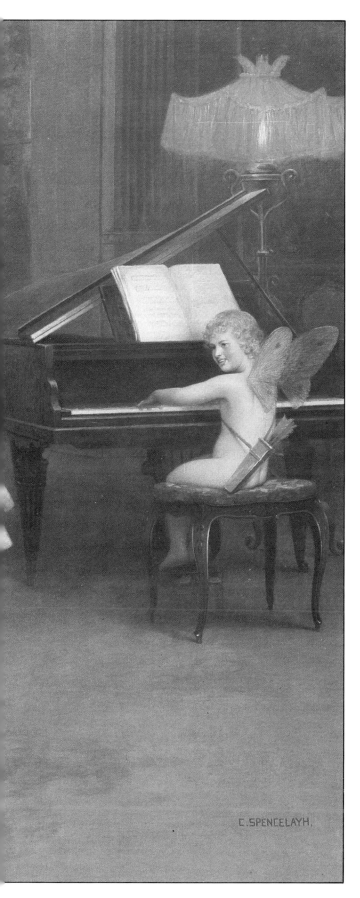

C.SPENCELAYH.

It was a hard time for blondes; the men of the Victorian era thought that the sexiest thing on four legs let alone two was a Steinway, and spent hours exorting their wives to make frilly pantaloons for those erotic little mahogany piano legs so that they did not become too inflamed at the sight of them sticking out just asking for it.

What kind of a time was this to be a woman, let alone a blonde?

When you looked behind the cushions on the sofa, or rooted in his drawers in the garden shed, all there was was dirty piano magazines showing various foreign makes in states of undress. What chance had women got against this potent sexual object?

None. Not even with the assistance of Harlene's Hair Products.

But while the Englishman was hanging valiantly on to his combinations, the French were still pondering the unanswerable question. *Why do gentlemen prefer blondes?* In 1886 Augustin Galopin wrote his magnum opus, *Le Parfum de Femme*, which was a book entirely based on the theory that women with different hair colours smell different. According to Augustin, who spent weeks sniffing around women in the interests of research, blondes had the odour of amber or violets. Something wrong there. If you think writing a book about blonde hair is a flimsy excuse, read his book!

Cupid plays a rousing selection from Rachmaninoff, while the young suitor, his loins pulsing with an ungovernable longing, proposes to his lady love. But! she wonders, but, but a thousand buts... should I tell him I was once voted Miss Texas Tomato, and perhaps lose his love forever?
Called Problem Paintings, this genre was enormously popular in Victorian times.

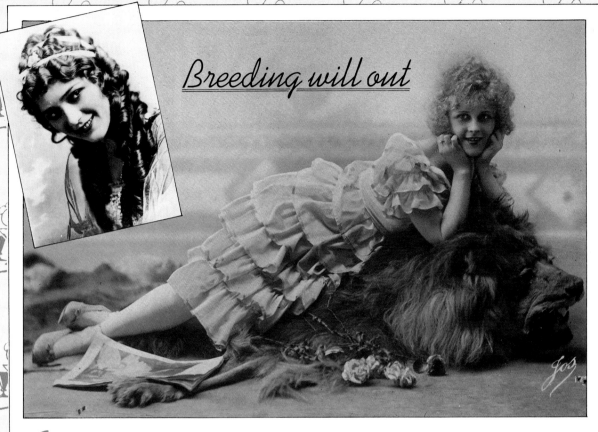

Breeding will out

One of the great literary hits of the 1920s, along with Michael Arlen's evocative tale *The Green Hat* (I say evocative because actually I haven't got further than page twenty-eight), was *Three Weeks* by Elinor Glyn. The heroine of this controversial romance endures – nay, enjoys – many moments of savage kisses and strained trouser fabric in front of a log fire. She lies in abandoned disarray on a tiger-skin rug, setting the pattern for great novels of the Twenties ...

When the story was filmed it was one of Hollywood's great brunettes, Gloria Swanson, who enjoyed the agonies and the ecstasies on the fevered set. No blonde actress could ever have played THAT heroine.

During the Twenties blondes followed the lead of the Cupid-like Mary Pickford who, with her husband Douglas Fairbanks, ruled Hollywood society like royalty. They threw endless soirées at their home, 'Pickfair', and Mary enjoyed her real-life role as America's sweetheart.

Following in her wake were a number of other blonde actresses with similar sausage curls and peaches-and-cream complexions – like Dorothy and Lillian Gish, Paulette Goddard and Marion Davies, who although fairly hopeless on screen had the advantage of being Randolph Hurst's girlfriend. This meant she was able to invite everyone back to his place for tea.

Then there were the bathing beauties like Bebe Daniels and Marie Prevost, who interestingly enough met her doom a few years later when she was eaten by her pet dog. And bringing up the rear in more ways than one were the brunette temptresses with exotic names and almond eyes: Pola Negri, Theda Bara and Swanson.

A curious thing hits me whenever I watch documentaries like 'Hollywood' on the telly. The women who starred in these early films chat away about the good year they had in 1923. BUT THEY ALL LOOK ABOUT FORTY-FIVE. Something is amiss; obviously Roman Polanski isn't the first director who should have had his legs slapped. Child molesting seems to have been rife. Most of these women must have starred in films at the age of fifteen and then married their directors a year later.

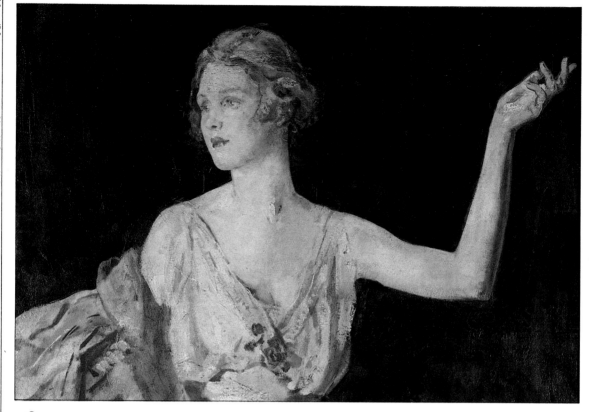

*I*n Britain there was an equally clearly defined social ladder and enjoying their view from the top of it were two great beauties: Barbara Cartland and Lady Diana Cooper. It seems doubtful that these two grandes dames would have been chums in their youth. Lady Diana, from the moment she could arrange her face into a pout, was a decadent, mysterious and enchanting figure. Barbara Cartland, while not renowned for exquisite beauty, was fending off the forty-eight proposals of marriage she received before she met Mr Right and writing a society gossip column (for £5 a week).

Some sixty years later, I told Lady Diana about Miss Cartland's legendary forty-eight proposals, only to receive a snort of derision for my trouble.

During my tea with her I became increasingly aware that in my efforts to agree with her, I was beginning to act like a model of Twi Twi in the back of a station wagon, nodding my head up and down like a yoyo.

Lady Diana lives in a white house in Little Venice, aptly decorated throughout with trompe l'oeil marble and portraits of herself and her mother, including one painted by Queen Victoria. Her lavatory is decorated with old royal Christmas Cards and on a table lay a letter addressed to her old friend the Queen Mother at Clarence House. The envelope was enlivened with red hearts and had I LUV YOO printed across the bottom, alongside what appeared to be one of Miss Cartland's cupids on a day off from holding up her begonias.

The Queen Mother had visited Lady Diana for lunch the week before. Minutes before her arrival, Lady Diana told me, chaos had ensued after she had glanced out of her window to discover THERE WERE NO ROSES TO BE SEEN in the garden. Quick as a flash she leapt into her Mini and drove to the Edgware Road, where she bought armfuls of plastic ones 'which I simply stuck into the stalks so it didn't look so bare'.

Lady Diana's mater was equally unconventional and equally beautiful. She appeared to be having such fun all the time that Edward VII took it upon himself to have words with her on the topic. A woman in her position, he told her, 'ought to drop cards and drive round and round Hyde Park in a barouche, and not go to supper parties, and draw and do amusing things.' Unfortunately as he reached the dignified close of his pep-talk the chair he was sitting on finally gasped its last breath and succumbed to the incessant nibbling of a herd of woodworms. He was pitched forwards onto the floor at Violet's feet.

In the words of Cecil Beaton, Diana is 'immortal, her name will go down with those of Helen, Cleopatra, Emma Hamilton and all the great Goddesses of Beauty.' After photographing her in Venice he noted: 'Her face is a perfect oval, her lips japonica red, her hair flaxen and her eyes are blue love-in-the-mist.' However, another slightly less besotted viewer commented simply, 'Her eyes were thrush-blue and she had a meditative trick of picking her nose while she was thinking.'

Rumours abounded about Diana. She wouldn't kiss boys in the back of taxis but one admirer gave her a mink all the same, which was henceforth referred to as 'the coat of shame'.

There are several problems inherent in meeting Miss Cartland. At all times you must remember to sit up straight, not to swear, to speak clearly and not to smoke. The latter rule apparently caused Lord Snowdon such distress when he went to photograph her that every time she left the room he could be found hovering around the fireplace puffing clouds of smoke up the chimney. If you want to write notes while she gives her views on the meaning of life, there are even more hurdles, for Miss Cartland cannot bear the sound of a pen scratching on paper, nor can she abide anyone using the last few pages of their notepad.

A white Rolls-Royce picks you up at the station when you are summoned to afternoon tea chez Cartland. As I was driven up the drive my face felt like it had been scrubbed with a brillo pad, I had washed so much. Ahead of me rose a vision – Miss Cartland's house resembles Buckingham Palace, if you can stretch your imagination to encompass Buck House meets Heidi. Amidst the soaring classical lines is the odd Tyrolean-style turquoise-blue shutter.

As Miss Cartland swept across the hall, which is about the same size as Shea Stadium, I was quick to notice that her dress and eyeshadow perfectly matched her paintwork. She paused by a gilded cupid holding aloft a large bowl of plastic begonias and waited for her pekinese, Twi Twi. The chauffeur leaned forwards and warned me not to touch Twi Twi in case he removed my hand.

Miss Cartland believes that the reason men don't propose with quite the alacrity they used to is because they think: 'Why buy a cow when you can milk it?' If nothing else she would have agreed wholeheartedly with Diana Cooper's back-seat embargo. Nor does she approve of the smuttier genre of romantic novels, where dire deeds are committed between the tooled plastic covers with raised gold lettering: 'They're disgusting. I bought a few of those novels at the station in Inverness, which you'd expect to be quite a respectable place. I thought they were revolting, I've never met women who behave like that. When a woman is in love she wants to feel it is sacred, not all that filthy carry-on.'

Diana Cooper married Duff, her unfortunately-named husband, in a flurry of great romance. Perhaps 'Duff' only refers to his poetical efforts – he wrote this to his wife:

Fear not, sweet love, what time can do,
Though silver dims the gold
Of your soft hair, believe that you
Can change but not grow old.

Duff was bewitched by Diana and fully understood that Evelyn Waugh, Randolph Churchill and others should wish to perch on the edge of her duvet to gaze in awe.

In a book called *Famous Women Reveal Their Beauty Secrets*, she told the nation hers: 'Lady Diana Receives in Bed'. The Bed soared sixteen feet into the air; from a shoal of golden dolphins and tridents, blue satin cascaded behind her and admirers wallowing in unrequited love must have thought they'd died and gone to heaven.

In her home in Maida Vale, Diana now has a buttercup-yellow bed. She has been

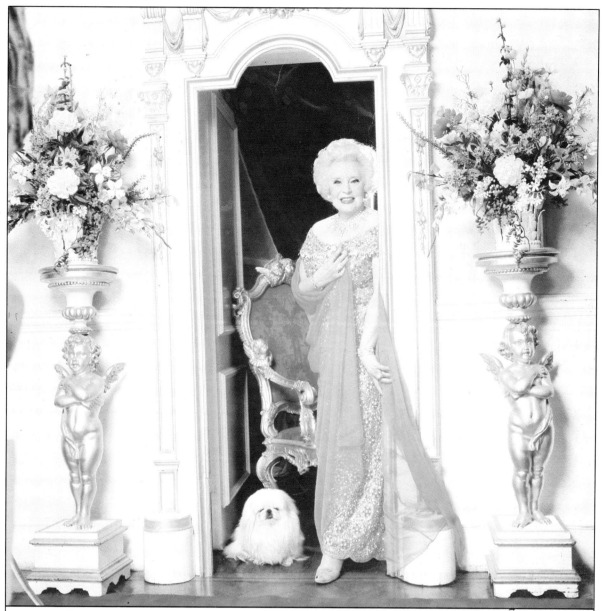

Capturing the essence of blondeness, Barbara Cartland and the blonde accessory – a short fat dog named Twi Twi. La Pompadour would be proud of the golden cupids and plastic begonias.

tied up on it several times by burglars, obviously after the coat of shame. Her little chihuahua, 'Doggie', cannot be of any great assistance during these burglaries, for his back leg has a tendency to drop out of its socket if he's kissed too hard, let alone given a rough-and-tumble with one of London's criminal classes.

Barbara Cartland is now the best-selling authoress in the world, and at one time it seemed that Diana Cooper was destined for true Hollywood stardom. She was the envy of the acting profession because of her ability to captivate audiences while standing stock still up a plinth for the first forty-six minutes of the play 'The Miracle'. After those soul-stiffening forty-six minutes she would descend from her eyrie to take on a nun's duties and clothes. One actress was so ferociously jealous of Diana that on the opening night she nailed the nun's veil to the stage. Diana descended to put the veil on and had to tug at it like a maddened terrier to get it off the floor.

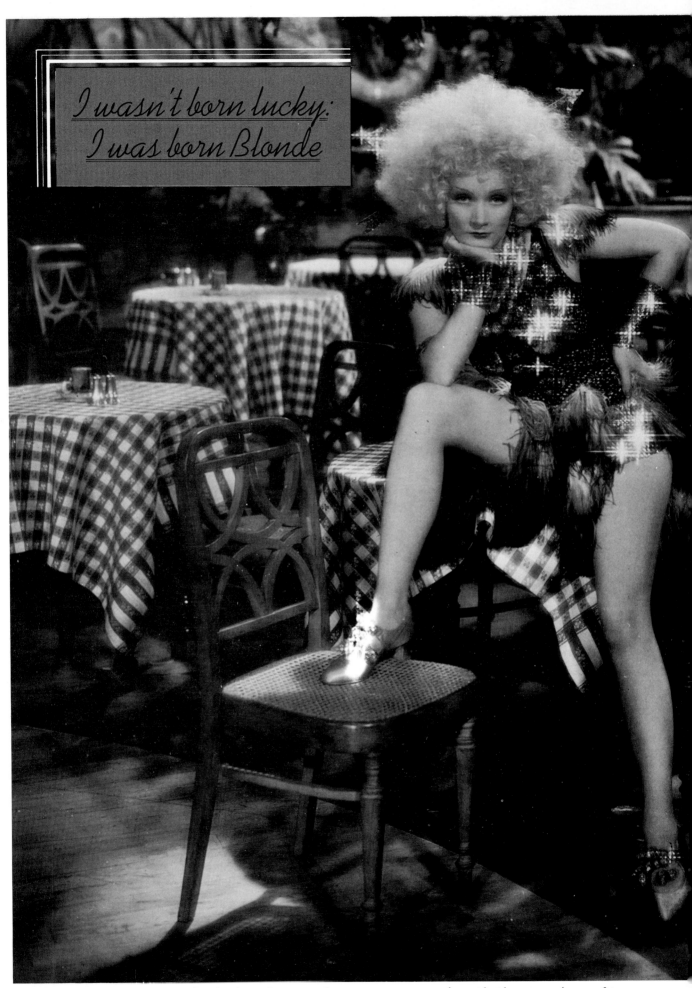

I wasn't born lucky: I was born Blonde

While Jean Harlow and Marlene Dietrich were concerned with their cooking, Veronica Lake's peek-a-boo hairstyle was so popular during the war that in England new rules

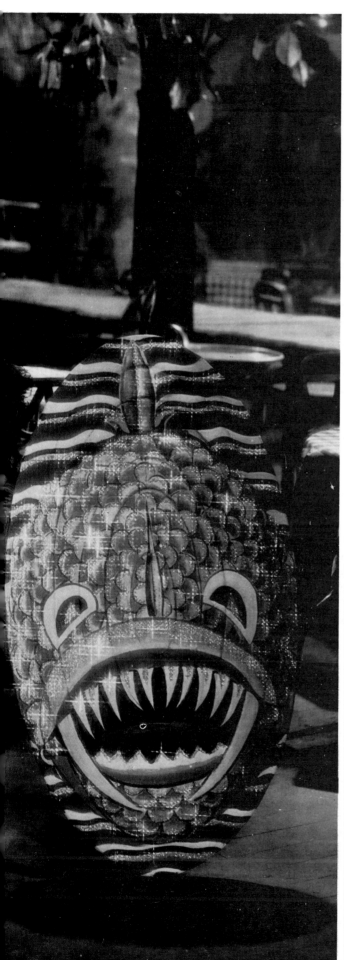

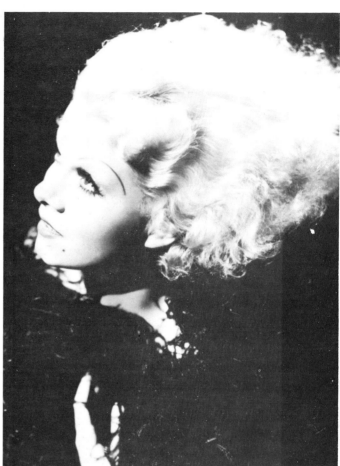

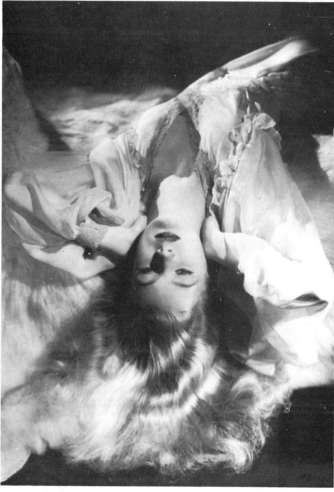

vere announced forbidding girls to have droopy gilt fringes on the factory floor. Girls had almost been garotted practising their pouts too close to machinery.

Mae West

*L*ater in life, when she began to be asked how she managed to stay looking so young, Mae West claimed that her secret was a daily enema. This was good enough fodder to silence those cruel beings who had imagined that Miss West in fact sellotaped large wodges of double chin behind her ears and then covered the whole lot up with cartwheel hats and ostrich feathers. Her penchant for white shagpile and young muscle-men with IQs never exceeding three, plus this daily enema, must have made her all-white home one of the few places in Hollywood during the Seventies where one could relive the Fall of the Roman Empire before eight.

Around 1972 I actually met Miss West in all her glory, complete with a cartwheel hat with a dead animal and several wax fruits perched on the top of it. She stunned the Universal Studios commissary in Hollywood into a respectful silence, as everyone craned their necks to see what she was going to eat. She had chicken broth. Some people strained to see if she was in drag, as a producer had once commented that she'd actually been playing the leading man all through her career.

West has always had a tendency to look like a drag queen on a night out, and her form of comedy – the innuendo-ridden, nudge-inducing variety – adds to the flavour. It was the nudging that got her into trouble first in 1926.

Mae had the bad luck to open her play – cosily entitled *Sex* – during a year when the Mayor 'Holy Joe' McKee was garnering votes with a clean-up campaign. Looking like an oversequinned, oversexed bratwurst as she wriggled across the stage, she socked it to packed audiences. Sadly she appears to have socked it to them too hard as she was promptly hauled in on a morals charge.

This is where Holy Joe's problems started and Mae West's infinite talent in the art of innuendo was proved. Nothing remotely obscene could actually be found in the play and the charges naturally began to shiver if not actually crumble. The District Attorney claimed that her 'personality, looks, walk, mannerisms and gestures made the lines and situations suggestive' – which is of course what the fun-starved Depression audiences were after. Here was a wonderful sexy Venus who made you laugh at sex not worry about it; she was a camp parody of all the sex goddesses who'd made sex seem like the Olympics.

The arresting officer corroborated what the attorney had said by rather graphically claiming that Miss West had 'moved her navel up and down and from left to right', leading many who read reports of the case to believe that the play included a steamy belly-dancing scene.

But during a Perry-Mason-like cross examination the officer, red-faced and obviously confused about anatomy in general, cracked under the strain. He admitted he'd not actually seen her navel, but something 'in her middle which moved from east to west'. Audiences never got to cram themselves into the theatre to try and spot what exactly was the nature of Mae West's wandering appendage. She was convicted and sentenced to ten days in jail. She served eight, with two days off for good behaviour.

In her main seven years on the big screen (where she seems to have had it stipulated in her contracts that she would only appear in films set in the Belle Epoque, giving her full rein to wear enormous bustles, corsets and the ubiquitous hat), she played liberated ladies who did the talking. In fact Mae had ALL the best lines, mainly because she wrote them. She squeezed every ounce of innuendo and anything else available from lines like, 'I was snow-white . . . but I drifted', 'It's not the men in my life . . . but the life in my men that counts' – which must have been true of the real men in her life, as it certainly wasn't their ability to discuss Jung that was the attraction.

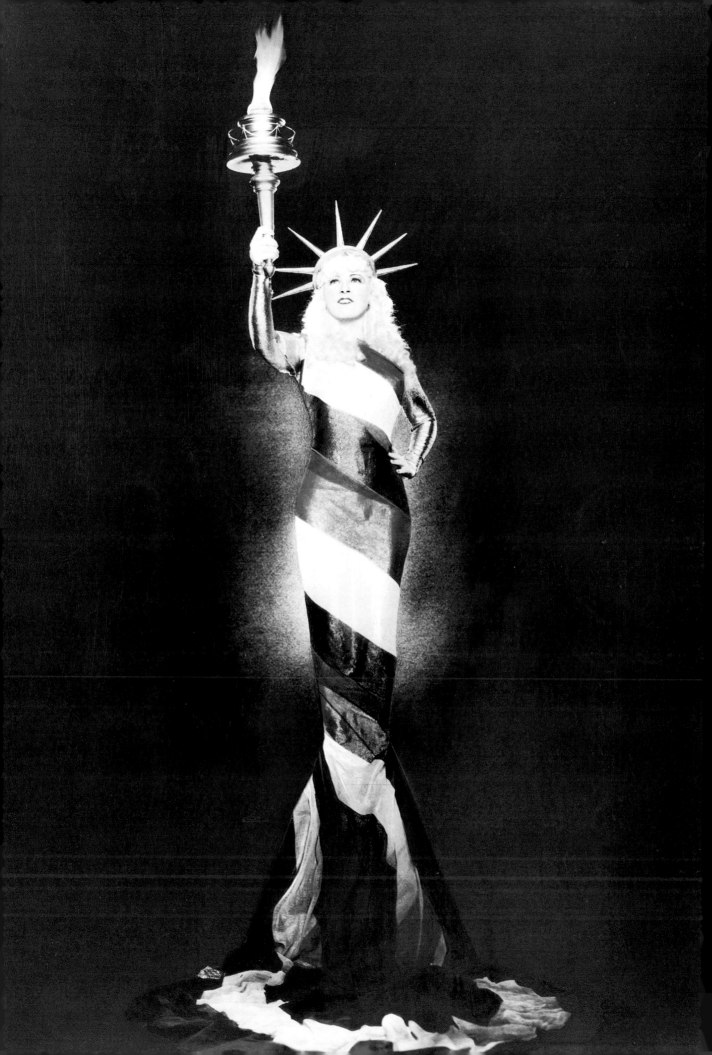

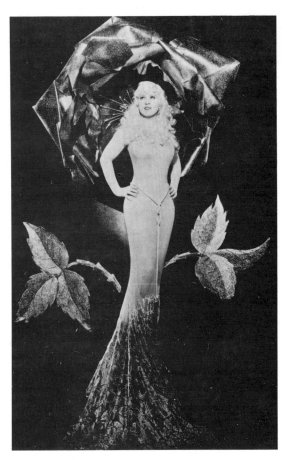

Shirley Temple

Shirley was the Thirties answer to Brooke Shields without the eyebrows and thighs. Both had forceful mothers hovering around on the set, and both became dolls – literally. There were ribbons, soap and lookalike competitions, with hundreds of squalling sprogs with the same fifty-six-curl hairstyle that Shirley sported.

Unfortunately what may have looked quite delightful on Shirley, with her cherubic face, looked less successful on your average six-year-old with a startling resemblance to Clive James.

The first words uttered by the incredibly edible Miss Temple on screen were, surprisingly, in French. '*Mais oui, mon cher,*' she squealed in *War Babies* – a satire on *What Price Glory?* Her other roles consisted mainly of match-making: Shirley Temple in the course of her musical career put together more couples than Dateline. She was also orphaned regularly and scored 200 on the CUTE-O-METER singing and dancing and showing her frilly knickers. And she did a mean imitation of Marlene Dietrich, as Morelegs Sweetrick – 'I wore lots of blue feathers and sequins, which I considered really dreamy. That's probably the most sirenish outfit I've ever worn on screen,' she later remarked.

Richard Watts noted in the *New York Herald* that, 'Although she is permitted to do some things that verge dangerously on the precocious, she never once made you want to spank her.'

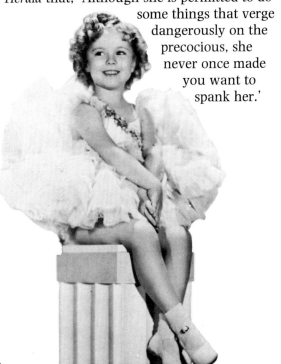

Her other good lines included classics like, 'When I'm good I'm very very good – but when I'm bad I'm even better' and the infamous, 'Is that a gun in your pocket or are you just pleased to see me?' – thus establishing herself, along with Harlow and Lombard, as one of the first women on screen to have the image of not needing men, just enjoying them.

In 1936 Mae was banned from appearing on the radio, no mean feat for someone whose sex appeal was meant to be based largely on swaggering and wiggling – neither of which come across very well on the radio. She was playing Eve, which leads one to wonder whether the casting director was drunk at the time, opposite Don Ameche as Adam and Edgar Bergen's dummy Charlie McCarthy as the snake. As she muttered, 'Would you ... (*pause*) ... honey ... like to try this apple?', the phones started buzzing ferociously, the fevers rose on the censors' brows and Mae's short-lived career in the biblical epic ended almost as soon as it had begun.

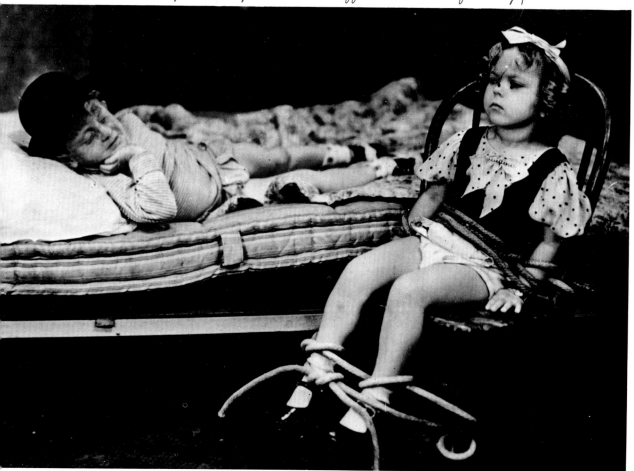

Dicky may have felt about her like this, but one of her co-stars, Adolphe Menjou, had different memories of starring opposite Shirley Temple:

> This child frightens me. She knows all the tricks. She backs me out of the camera, blankets me, crabs my laughs. She's making a stooge out of me. Why, if she was forty years old she wouldn't have had time to learn all the tricks she knows about acting. Don't ask me how she does it. You've heard about chess champions at eight, and violin virtuosos at ten. Well, she's Ethel Barrymore at six.

Rumours circulated that she was in fact a midget and that trick photography was used to keep her looking eternally small and youthful. I know how she felt. I was once judging a competition when a young boy with acne wandered up to me and asked, 'Do they use trick photography on you on telly?' 'No,' I replied shortly. 'Why?' He took a step back to peruse every inch of me. 'Well, it's just that you're a right dog in the flesh,' he told me before returning to his pint.

In 1934, after the eighth Shirley Temple release of the year, she was presented with a special Oscar. Members of the Academy fresh from seeing Shirley's rendition of 'On the Good Ship Lollipop' in *Bright Eyes* announced that it was 'for bringing more happiness to millions of children and millions of grown-ups than any child of her years in the history of the world'. She also got to place her footsteps in the wet cement outside Grauman's Chinese Theater, preserved forever alongside the Hollywood greats.

Not everything ran smoothly for the dimpled moppet. When she was six her mother took her to see Santa Claus. She promptly stopped believing in him. 'The first thing he did,' she recalls, 'was ask for my autograph.'

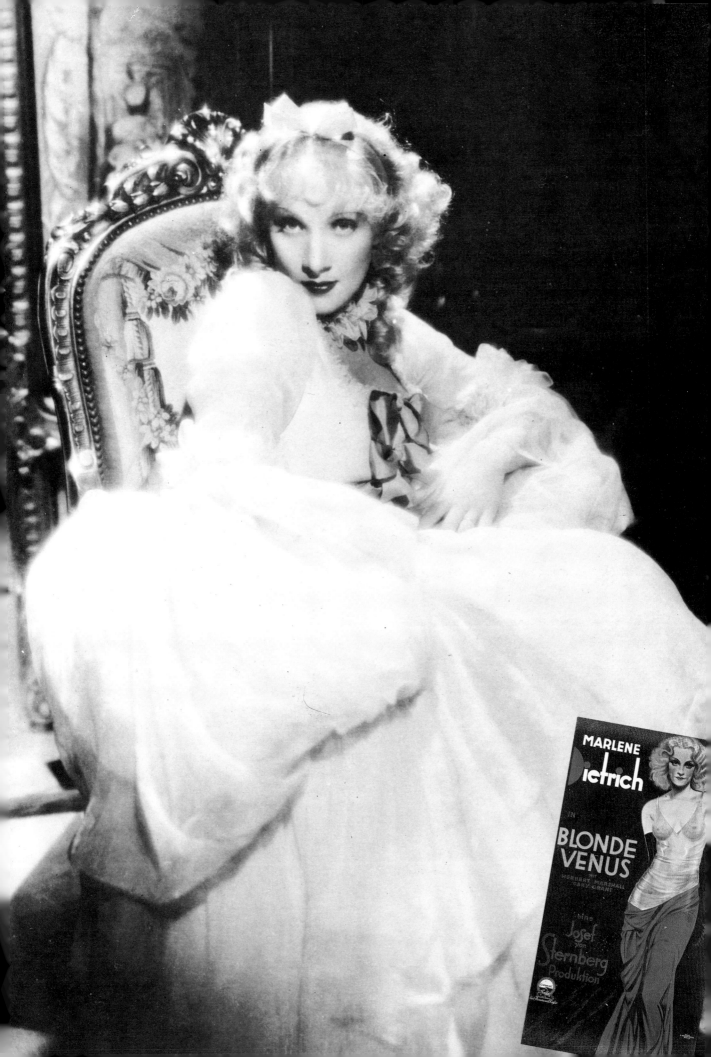

Marlene Dietrich

*M*arlene Dietrich was one of those lucky women with a Svengali. I would like one as soon as possible. I used to think that I got headaches from trying to see things without my specs on, but now I realise I get headaches from trying to think. I want someone else to do that for me. Send John Derek anytime. I'd love a boyfriend who snatched the wine-gums out of my mouth in the cinema...

Despite her appearance in Hollywood during the Forties as a female wolf in men's clothing, underneath her men's suits she was Josef von Sternberg's little lambikins. Contrary to the severe look she cultivated, Marlene barely blew her nose without Josef first making sure that she looked okay while she did it. He was the man who discovered her while she was still a little plump girl. The great thing about all Svengalis is their ability to spot sirens underneath layers of puppy fat and blue eyeshadow.

This is how von Sternberg recalled their first meeting, when he was auditioning girls for his film, *Der Blaue Engel*: 'I sent her to the wardrobe to discard her street clothes and she returned wearing something roomy enough to contain a hippopotamus'.

Despite this she got the part and, after some persuasion from von Sternberg, Paramount made her an offer no one would refuse. She did. She wasn't sure that she wanted to leave her husband and her child in Germany and travel to Hollywood. It was only after the premiere that she gingerly decided to travel alone to the States.

Her first American film was to be *Morocco*, opposite Gary Cooper. Von Sternberg immediately forbade her to eat anything he hadn't vetted and had her pummelled madly by masseurs twice a day. She was also made up by experts who gave her pencilled-in eyebrows and made sure that her cheeks looked suitably consumptive. After all this effort she was then photographed peering myoptically through boughs, lace, fogs and the arches of convents.

By 1931 her husband and her daughter joined her in America and von Sternberg, by now nicknamed by the studio 'Svengali Joe', had her photographed with her little girl. It was the first time that any screen Goddess had been seen with her own child. But it was necessary because Dietrich simply couldn't resist displaying her domestic talents to every journalist who came to interview her. They would expect her to answer the door with a feather boa seductively shielding one eye: instead she would sweep to the door with a meat loaf. She would feed hacks up and send them home with the recipes.

After a while von Sternberg became thoroughly sick of all the old crappola that was being sent to him by the studio and wrote his own script for her – *Blonde Venus*. One of the most memorable scenes in the film is 'Hot Voodoo', a sort of jungle version of Jailhouse Rock which features Dietrich making her entrance somewhat incongruously clad in a gorilla suit. As she sways to the infernal pounding of jungle rhythms her hand maidens assist her out of her fur rug and she is handed a spear, shield and loincloth. The popularity of loincloths worn in the privacy of one's own home increased immediately.

Lana Turner

*T*here is no doubting that Lana is a lot better as a name for a hotsie than Jean Mildred, which were two of Turner's real names. She came by her exotic name through the simple act of spelling ANAL backwards. One wonders what her press agents had spent the rest of the meeting doing. Screwing up bits of paper with possibles written on them? Sally Turner, Holly Turner, Nancy Turner – NO, they shrieked, when finally a tall dark enraged press agent must have leapt to his feet and shouted 'If you don't decide soon you can spell anal backwards for all I care ...' and stormed out.

Lana had come to this historic moment of renaming by a number of other legendary moments, starting when she was discovered by the editor of *Hollywood Reporter* making farting noises down the straw in her milk shake. Billy Wilkerson sidled over to her and said HOWDYA LIKETA BE IN PICTURES?

Shwabbs, the icecream parlour where the meeting is supposed to have occurred, has never had it so good since then. Every would-be Francis Ford Coppola and Marilyn Monroe sits in there waiting to be discovered.

No thickie, Lana merely laughed nonchalantly in Mr Wilkerson's face before wriggling off to tell her Mater what had happened. She shrewdly paused on the way home to buy a copy of the *Hollywood Reporter* so that she could check his credentials before going to his office dressed up 'like a pup at a dog show'.

The first piece of advice she received was *Never overdress*. She went on to become Hollywood's first Sweater Girl in her first role, which called for her to walk seventy-five feet in possibly the tightest orlon knit in history. She looked like a creamy blonde volcano wrapped in angora. Lana didn't visualize herself this way off screen. She took her mother to see the film and was horrified when the entire cinema erupted at the sight of her and her bottom. Lana's bum seemed

to have a life all its own. During that seventy-five feet of pavement, it seemed to be following Lana three paces behind and jiggling furiously from the effort of keeping up. Mrs Turner sank lower and lower in her seat and Lana claims she didn't turn her back on anyone for weeks in case they spotted her rear end.

Despite the fact that her bottom made its debut before the rest of her, it was Lana's jumper that teenagers longed to copy.

Unlike many of her peers, who secretly longed to play Ibsen with themselves in all the roles, Lana never once longed to let her glamorous façade slip. Not for her the Oscar for getting fat or the Oscar for not wearing make-up in a film. Lana was always impeccably groomed and glacially cool even if she was meant to be in the midst of an emotional holocaust.

The only time that audiences ever got to see Lana in an emotional state was in real life, when she was called to the witness box after her daughter Cheryl Crane stabbed Lana's dodgy gangland boyfriend. Not only did Lana have to testify, her steamy letters to Johnny Stompanato where all over the front pages. If Lana were to start her career

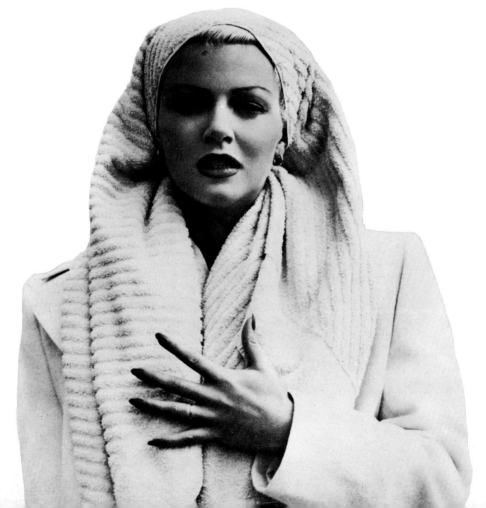

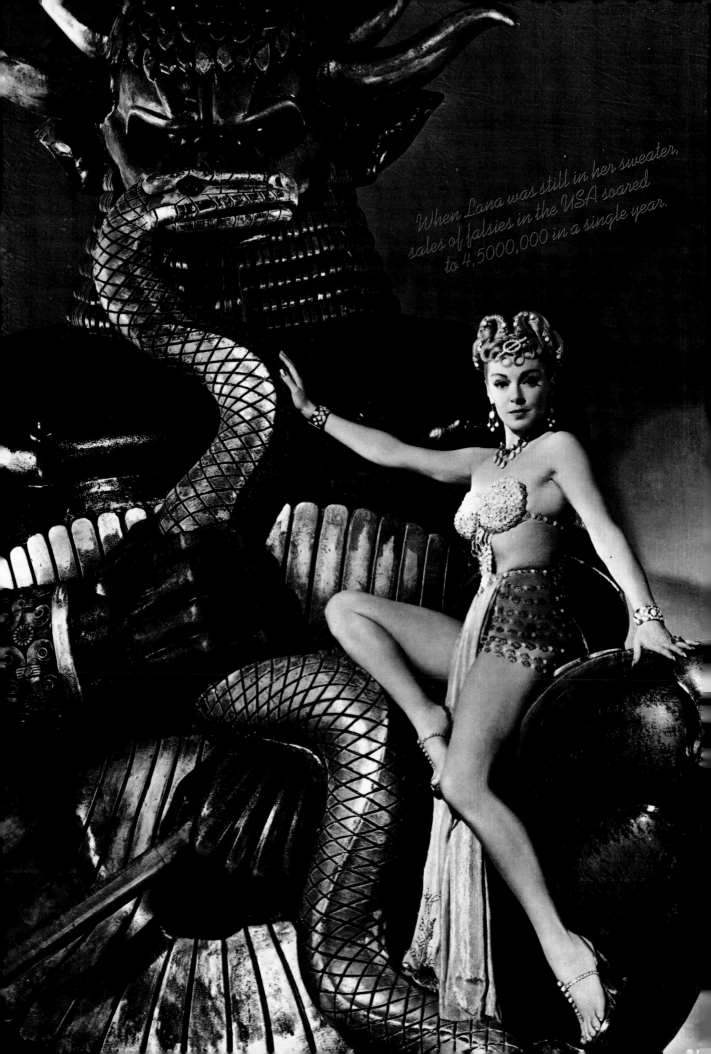

When Lana was still in her sweater,
sales of falsies in the USA soared
to 4,5000,000 in a single year.

over again, her line in purple prose would make romantic novels an obvious choice of job. She would take to writing about throbbing iron-hard manhoods like a duck to water.

Instead Lana's later career was soap operas, although her private life always had the better story lines.

She was in *Peyton Place* (that haven for blondes) alongside Mia Farrow, who caused headlines every time she got a haircut, and Ryan O'Neal. Now Miss Turner is in 'Falconcrest', an American dynastic number where she appears to be the secret unknown mother of almost every male member of the cast. The entire point of 'Falconcrest' is that each week it is revealed that Lana Turner is someone else's mother.

Her fans always claim that her greatest role was in *The Postman Always Rings Twice*, as the murderous wife. Not for her any rolling around on the kitchen table. In Lana's version, the sight of her lipstick case rolling across the floor and then the camera panning almost up the leg of her shorts was enough to have audiences reeling with its orgasmic significance.

Betty Grable

When the raw materials you're working on look like Hammy the Hampster with his cheeks filled with nuts for the winter, it's obvious that the things to publicize lie far beneath these protruberances.

Studio publicists decided to give Betty Grable million-dollar legs rather than the million-dollar chops which she could also have aspired to. These famed legs (7½-inch ankle, 12-inch calves and 18½-inch thighs) set pulses racing. The campaign worked. By 1934 she was the Number One box-office star and she remained firmly on that list until 1953.

Her poster, which showed her from the rear with her backside poked firmly in the GIs' direction, sold two million copies. Not that Grable had any pretensions whatsoever about herself or her appeal:

Of course I'm strictly an enlisted man's girl. I do not mean that I do not like officers or that officers do not like me. But I am a truck-driver's daughter and so I have got to be an enlisted man's girl, just like this has got to be an enlisted man's war. A lot of these kids don't have any women in their lives to fight for and I guess what you would call us girls is kind of their inspiration. It is a grave responsibility.

A few of the films that Betty appeared in made her seem less than muse-like. At first she was put into a few black-and-white films until a Fox executive decided, wisely, that Grable looked better in living, not to say livid, colour. 'Her hair and skin are perfect for this kind of presentation,' he explained, 'and when she waves her hips in a colour film she does it a favour.'

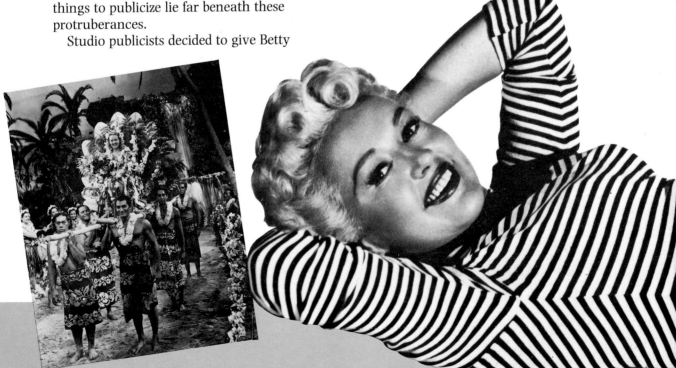

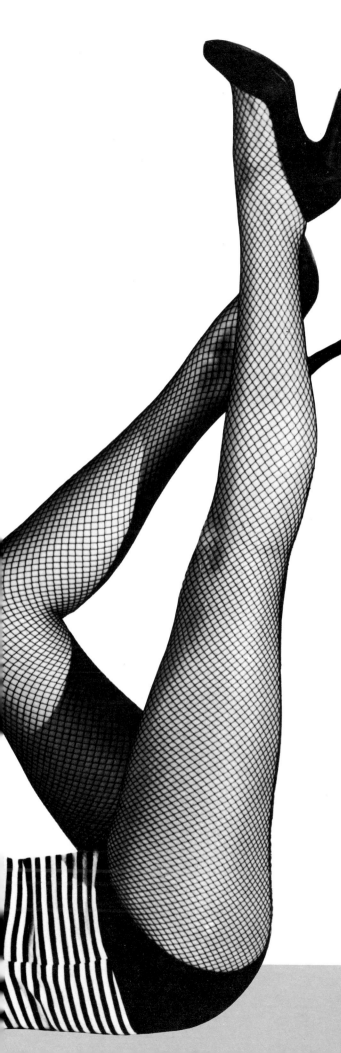

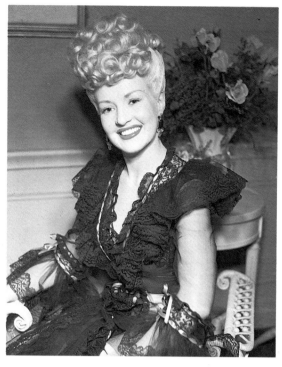

One of the epics in which her hips did the most waving and everyone else forgot about acting almost entirely was *Song of the Islands* – a slightly improbable tale of an Irish beachcomber's daughter, with Victor Mature as the love interest who gets swept up on the beach as she combs it. The film now looks like a promotional video for gay clubs in the Bay Area, with endless strings of big boys in arran jumpers doing the splits behind Betty.

The film provided the world with songs like '*O'Brien has gone Hawaiian*' and the interestingly entitled '*Down on Ami Ami Oni Oni Isle*'. Not that Betty was any newcomer to songs like that. One of my favourite lines of all time is from *Lady In Ermine* where she sings straightfaced, 'Ooooo what I'll doooo to that wild Hungarian.' Luckily Betty never had any desire to play the classics and was more interested in her family and the race-track than any of these films!

Grable met Rory Calhoun during the filming of *How to Marry a Millionaire*. She was starring with Marilyn Monroe, that decade's blonde. Rory played a stupid forest ranger. Obviously he was a dumb ranger with other strings to his bow. In 1969, Betty was named in his divorce case along with seventy-eight other women.

Great Blonde Fascists of our Time

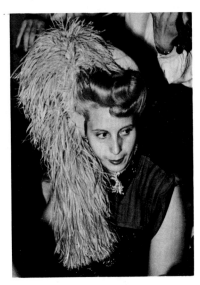

With another General Election just behind us it will be interesting to see whether Saatchi and Saatchi ever nick any ideas from the past. Shirley Williams could get a whole new lease of life from some of Eva Peron's political ruses. Instead of the slogans like 'Labour Doesn't Work', voters would finally get what they're after with 'SHIRL GIVES BETTER BLOW JOBS' writ large across the nation. Eva Peron's talent for this activity was always more widely whispered about when an election drew close or if she needed extra support to push one of her ideas through government. It's probably only because of the difficulty in finding a rhyme for job that it wasn't mentioned in the musical.

And while the people of Britain were still reeling from Shirley's candid revelation, she could fling her Paddington-Bear-at-a-1963-CND-rally outfit into the bin. Instead of the jumpers hand-knitted out of muesli, Shirley could arrive at a few all-night sittings with the plumes of a bird of paradise cascading flirtily over one eye, as Eva often did.

Eva Peron's own rise to power (albeit by proxy, via Juan) is made all the more astonishing if one contemplates the average South American's grasp of women's rights. In the immortal words of Barbie Cartland the reply would be, 'Rights, what rights?'

In her unquenchable desire for power Eva reversed the blonde's usual Svengali syndrome.

Eva Peron was Juan Peron's John Derek. Astutely she realized that Argentinians would not accept a woman in control, so her image carefully made her look as frivolous and safe as possible. Under her floaty silk chiffons beat a heart that made Mrs Thatcher look like a nancy.

Her campaign posters, which were plastered everywhere, were painted to look like the religious pictures of the time, slightly blurred, very garish and heavily touched up. She was like a movie star rather than a politician as she gazed benevolently down, blonde hair swept up and moist red lips slightly parted. I can see it now at the next Election – Shirl on a chaise longue in a silk peignoir. It's the sort of thing that would turn anyone SDP.

Eva was a million miles away from her youth at this point. She grew up poor, illegitimate and, worse still for her ambitions, totally flat-chested. But her stay in power wasn't destined to last long. She died of cancer when she was thirty-three. Oddly Juan decided to have her body embalmed and preserved (YUK). It was a big mistake. Even in death Eva was dogged by bad luck. Her body was nicked from its resting place with alarming regularity. It doesn't even bear thinking what people wanted it for. Eventually it was rumoured that her body had travelled more miles while she was dead than while she was alive. Finally she came to rest, but all those pilferings had wrought havoc on her. Eva Peron's body was found to have shrunk to the size of a frail twelve-year-old. Only her hair remained its old rich lustrous gold.

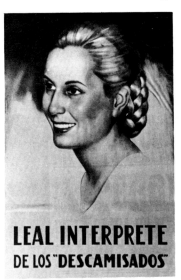

More blow jobs – more votes?

LEAL INTERPRETE
DE LOS "DESCAMISADOS"

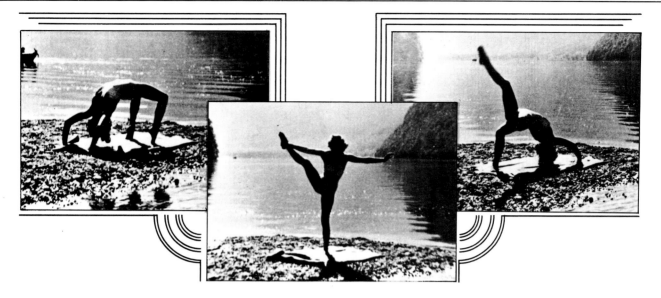

One of the few women who have lived up to the myth of the blonde as a person who is beautiful, youthful, innocent and thick as two short planks was Eva Braun. Eva Prawn would have been more like it. Eva was young, lovely, long-legged and had absolutely nothing on her mind except keeping the Führer enchanted with his little bunny-wunny.

Her blondeness must have helped. Hitler's ideal aryan, as represented in fascist posters of the time, resembled adverts for a new gay nightclub. Even more dubious is how a short fat Austrian with greasy dark hair planned to become the leader of this nation of superhuman elitist blondes with thighs like iron.

Eva was very devoted. She referred to herself as 'the mistress of Germany's – and the world's – greatest man', which must have pleased him if he ever took the time to rummage in her knicker drawer for the diaries. It was this sort of thing, which she would say without guile, that charmed the pants off Hitler.

Eva wasn't allowed to go to the great state dinners. Instead she was hostess at the small parties given for heads of state in private at Hitler's mountain-top retreat, Berghof. She was mistress of Berghof and spent almost all her time there. Much to Hitler's relief. He had told many people that she was an aristocrat, and would spend hours boasting of his girlfriend's noble family. This ruse would have been entirely ruined had anyone met her. For all her charm, Eva by reports was apt to overdress horribly and never quite forgot her working-class background.

She would spend hours changing from one swimsuit to another, exercising, making films of herself doing the exercises and then editing them so that any bits where she fell on her bum were left on the cutting-room floor. Eva was very pre-aerobics and can be seen in these films with legs flapping wildly, going for the burn like a forerunner of those repellent Californian types in salmon-pink leotards looking like freshly squeezed liver sausages. Eva makes it all seem more like Grumping Iron than Pumping Iron. The films show her as she spent her days alone, playing with kittens, diving and dancing. One of the racier ones shows her sister Greta and a number of other nubile young German girls all naked under a waterfall.

Despite his enjoyment of these examples of Cinema Vérité, Hitler's great ambition was to change all of Eva's frivolous habits. These, it has to be said, were legion. Stopping Eva's compulsive shopping caused him more headaches than wiping out entire races.

Almost everything that he considered pure and pristine she considered boring and dull. He never ate meat, smoked or drank, whereas she 'wolfed down steaks, ignoring his disapproval,' according to the housekeeper. She also chain-smoked and drank whisky. Worse still, when Hitler treated himself to a cup of herb tea after a busy day at the office, Eva would be in her boudoir quaffing a pint mug of champagne which she claimed, not really surprisingly, 'helped her to sleep'.

I like them fluffy I freely confess,
With fluffy blue eyes and a fluffy blue dress,
And fluffy fair hair and no brains at all.
A. P. Herbert

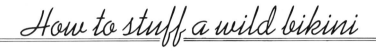

How to stuff a wild bikini

During the twentieth century, when our ideal blondes have been represented almost entirely by film stars, each new decade has brought another style of blonde. The Thirties had independent girls who laughed at sex. In the Forties, while the men were on the war front, the women back home were transformed into svelte sirens. The Fifties had a whole new breed of star.

The Fifties blonde was the girl to match the new utopia that postwar America was aspiring to. She was gossy, artificial and bigger than anything that had gone before, in every area of her anatomy except her brain. The Fifties may have boasted blondes with all the sheen of a newly sprayed Ford Cortina but they had none of the horse power.

These girls had something in common with the woman of that other Golden Age, the eighteenth century: they didn't like washing and were grubby with a very large G. The stars of the time may have dressed from head to toe in pure white – but underneath they were tide-marked. Don't believe Monroe when she said she wanted to be BLONDE ALL OVER.

Monroe and Mansfield were neither of them given to hours of abluting, in fact their idea of purgatory must have been those obligatory photo sessions under mounds of bubbles. Soap was to them what Le Corbusier is to modern architecture. A big mistake. Given that simile both of them would have cried, 'Bring back mock tudor all is forgiven.'

But one must be thankful for all mercies. Both of them had a horror of underwear. Had either of them worn knickers, it's safe to say they might have left them on for the entire decade as a celebration.

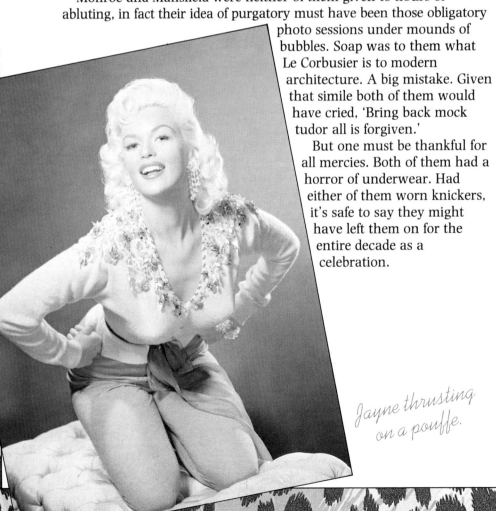

Jayne thrusting on a pouffe.

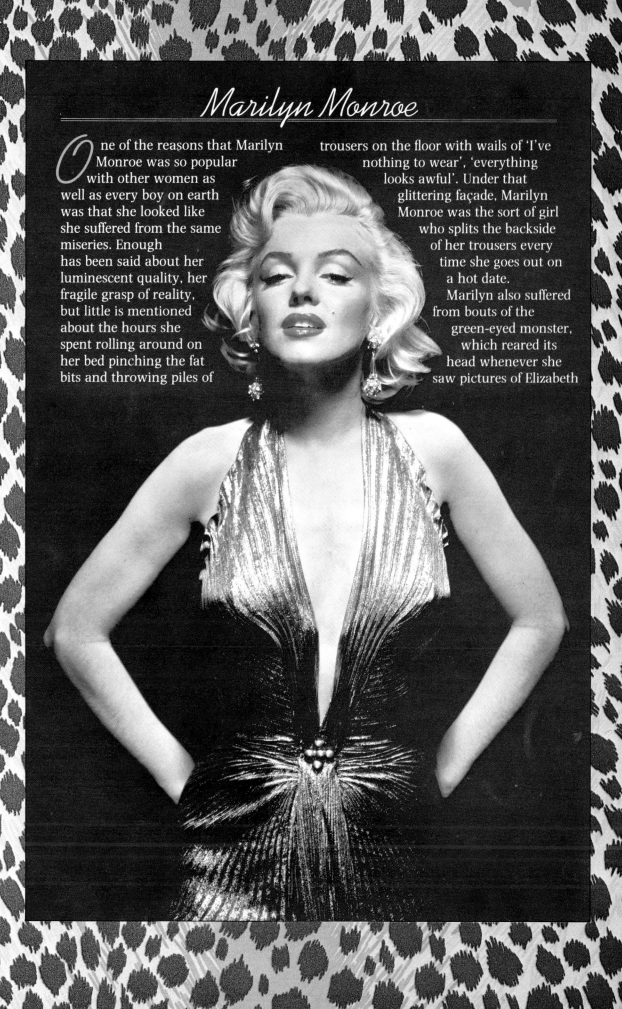

Marilyn Monroe

One of the reasons that Marilyn Monroe was so popular with other women as well as every boy on earth was that she looked like she suffered from the same miseries. Enough has been said about her luminescent quality, her fragile grasp of reality, but little is mentioned about the hours she spent rolling around on her bed pinching the fat bits and throwing piles of trousers on the floor with wails of 'I've nothing to wear', 'everything looks awful'. Under that glittering façade, Marilyn Monroe was the sort of girl who splits the backside of her trousers every time she goes out on a hot date.

Marilyn also suffered from bouts of the green-eyed monster, which reared its head whenever she saw pictures of Elizabeth

Taylor. Like most people who are a teensy-weensy bit jealous, she further fuelled this by buying every magazine with Taylor on the cover and then gloating over Taylor's fat fingers. Monroe is said to have been delighted to discover that Taylor bit her nails.

At one point she decided to seduce Montgomery Clift, which seems a reasonable thing to want to do. If he hadn't died, *I* would have proposed to him.

First, Marilyn convinced herself that he was sleeping with Liz Taylor. 'I bet Monty sleeps with her, I bet he does,' she'd say, adding miserably 'WHY HER?'

Marilyn had heard all the rumours that he was in fact a drug-addicted queen but for her the whole concept of two men sleeping together was too bizarre to even contemplate. 'Why would he do that?' she said, unable to visualize the ins and outs of it, when her friends tried gently to explain that he simply didn't like girls. 'He could have any woman he wanted.'

Marilyn's blind spot where homosexuality was concerned led to a hilarious afternoon spent plying the half-awake Clift with caviar and vodka. At the end of the afternoon she was inclined to agree with the old French tradition of refusing to give actors Christian burials.

Clift was asked round for tea and arrived several hours later, which gave Monroe more time to try on the rest of her wardrobe and split it. After sewing her trousers onto her, make-up artists and hairdressers prepared her for the big seduction.

Clift laid his head on her lap and she fed him the caviar with a silver spoon. She then slid her head into his unfortunately entirely lifeless lap. Her intimate looks and pulsating walks across the apartment were having less than no effect on him: he continued to

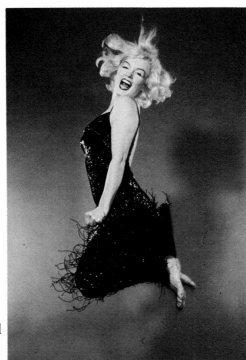

discuss all the different sleeping pills he'd tried, his new shrink and his part in *Freud*.

Finally, as a last-ditch attempt to turn his blood to molten lava, Marilyn wriggled across the room and stuck her bottom in his face as she bent over to pour him another vodka. He stood up. This is it, she gasped to herself.

'You've got the most incredible ass,' he said as he reeled towards her front door. 'But I gotta be going.'

As soon as the crumpet of the century had staggered out of the door Marilyn fell back onto the sofa and shrieked with laughter, admitting absolute defeat. She comforted herself with the thought that Liz Taylor couldn't possibly be doing it with him either. Then she disappeared into her bedroom where she spent the rest of the afternoon on the bed in the nude, listening to Frank Sinatra records and kissing his record sleeve, and day-dreaming of Clark Gable.

These two were real pals. Sinatra gave Marilyn a little French poodle which, much to his annoyance, she named Maf, short for Mafia. He told her that anyone knew a little poodle should have a suitably French name like Pierre. Gable starred with her in *The Misfits*, and his constant references to her as Chubbychops and Fatso sent her into ecstasies despite her chronic lack of self-confidence. When the scene finally came where he had to kiss her she was in heaven for several weeks, telling her girlfriends that this moment was 'like, like ... er ... like kissing Clark Gable'.

Monroe had a lot of odd habits at home. Like Carole Lombard before her, she dyed her pubic hair. Lombard had always referred to this athletic practice as 'keeping her collar and cuffs matching'. In order to dye the offending hair, Monroe would retire to the

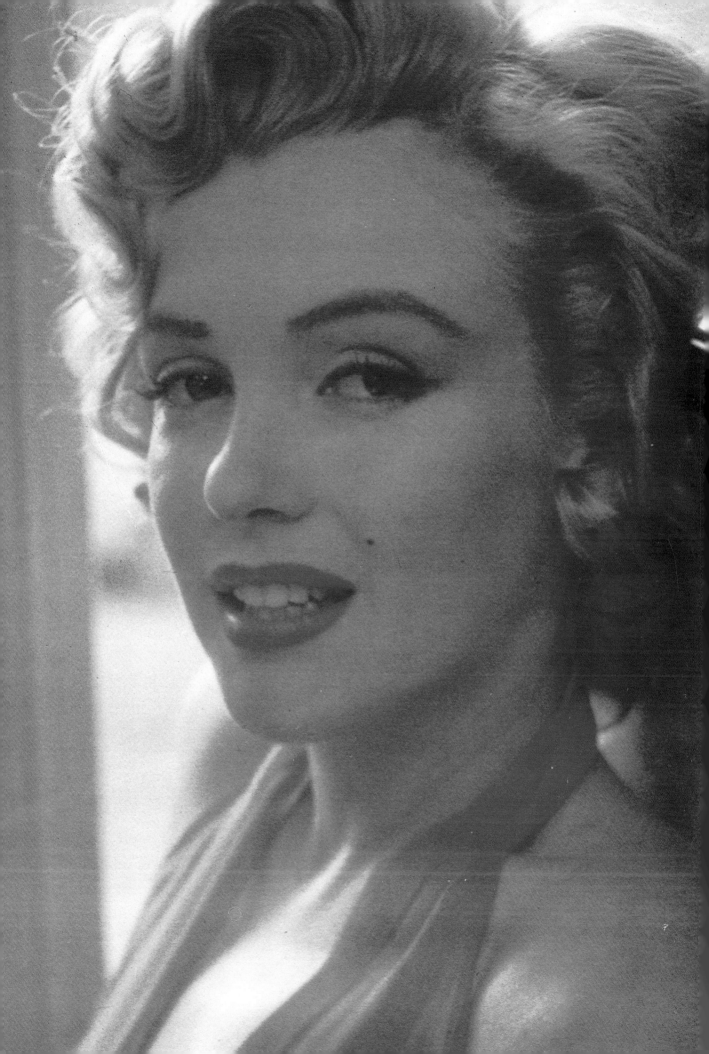

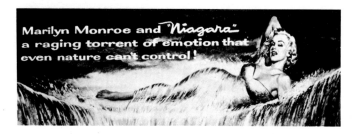
Marilyn Monroe and "Niagara" a raging torrent of emotion that even nature can't control!

bathroom armed with dye and a toothbrush. She'd then sit backwards on the loo with both legs waving in the air. But this home do-it-yourself technique often resulted in her getting the most painful infections which she treated with an icepack between her legs. Apart from this self-inflicted pain, the only other real illness from which Monroe suffered constantly came rather unromantically from her gall bladder. If she ate too much, which she frequently did, it made her fart and belch continuously which she found hilarious. According to her Italian cook she ate far too much: a typical day could include three eggs, toast, three plates of chips, veal cutlets, two chocolate milkshakes, three hamburgers, three plates of eggplant parmigiani, spaghetti, and four bowls of chocolate pudding to finish it all off. This was all washed down with lots of champagne in bed.

With a diet like that it's not surprising that Miss Monroe had severe problems with her flatulence.

Jayne Mansfield

Jayne Mansfield claimed throughout her career to have a stunning IQ of 160. She also sought throughout her career to make this statement as unbelievable as possible. Jayne acted as though her IQ would barely hit four-and-a-half on a hot day.

Her array of husbands – chosen mainly for their ability to give her a good smack in the face at regular intervals, wear leopard-print loincloths and do the grouting and plumbing on her heart-shaped swimming pool and fourteen bathrooms – are enough to convince anyone what a berk she was.

She even enjoyed her first film role, as a

dead body lying on a pavement in the aptly named *Hangover*. The film was being made on such a cheap budget that there was no extra cash to be spared on a stand-in or a dummy, so Jayne had to lie for hours in full make-up without moving a muscle in the blazing sun. Jayne decided that she might be dead in that film but underneath she was a sex goddess of A grade quality.

'I guess a lot of people think that a girl who shows her bosom and wears tight dresses can't be close to God. But God has always been very close to me,' Jayne told the press, adding, 'I have to look like a star 24 hours a day ... I'm always on, I get more press than Liz Taylor even.'

Jayne was certainly using her brains very secretly. She'd bought the infamous Pink Palace which, according to one wit, had 'a nice view overlooking the mortgage'. It possessed such desirable qualities as pink terraces, endless pink bathrooms with heart-shaped tubs, electrically-operated loo seats, gold and onyx swan-shaped taps, loo-roll holders with crinolines that played the Marseillaise when you lifted them and pink French-style telephones in every room. Jayne lived up to her home, everything about her turned pink. She strode down Sunset Boulevard with a Great Dane and a rented ocelot on a leash, both of them wearing pink satin bows. She arrived everywhere with an entourage of her endless babies (Jayne had five) and endless

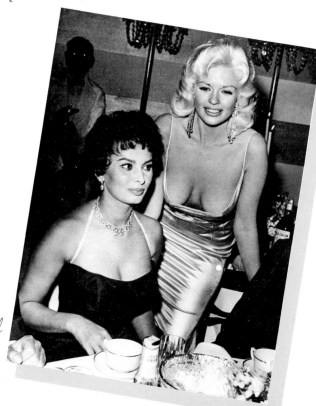
A moment of keen competition between Jayne and Sophia Loren. Sophia's mouth has temporarily gone like a chicken's bottom.

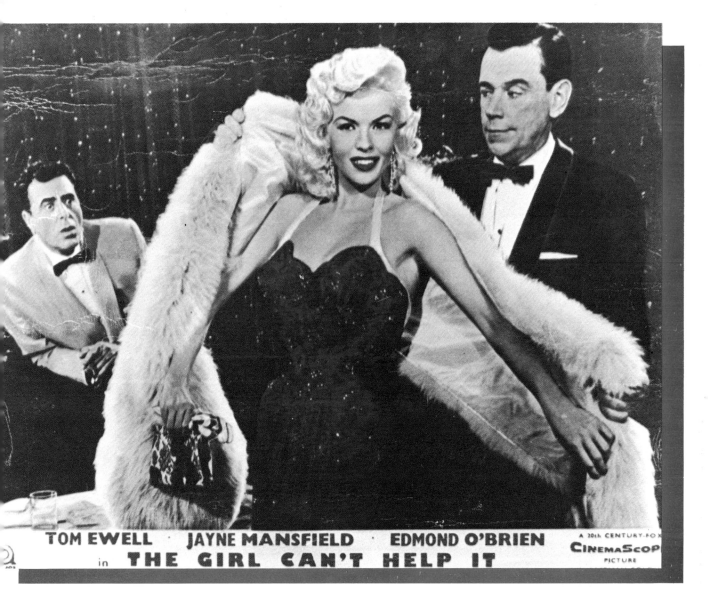

TOM EWELL · JAYNE MANSFIELD · EDMOND O'BRIEN
in THE GIRL CAN'T HELP IT

A 20th CENTURY-FOX
CINEMASCOP
PICTURE

puppies, and hotels thanked God that Jayne, with her apparent blind spot about housetraining, only *rented* the fucking ocelot.

Jayne had a romantic life that has never been equalled even by the heady standards of modern-day starlets. At fourteen she was raped and became pregnant. Sensibly she picked out the best-looking boy in her high school, lied about her age and got married. From then on she had children regularly and was always represented in the press as an ideal mother, despite the fact that they had to wade through dog shit to get to her.

'I'm too much woman not to get pregnant,' she cried.

Then Grace Kelly announced her engagement to Prince Rainier. Quick as a flash Jayne was speculating to the press about her own romantic ambitions: 'I want to marry royalty and have a crest on all my nightgowns too.'

A couple of days later she was at it again:

A woman loves to think of herself as a little kitten to be pampered and adored. I do, I'm twenty-three and eligible. I'd like to meet Bob Wagner, Bob Stack, Tyrone Power, Marlon Brando and Liberace, bless his heart. And somewhere I hope there's a real prince for me. I want LOTS of babies. I'm good and healthy, I want to become a Princess or even a QUEEN if there's a king for me.

Despite this, Jayne next settled for a Hungarian body-builder called Micky Hargitay. Mickey inspired Miss Mansfield to yet more announcements, her bulletins to the breathless Hollywood press came thick and fast.

'OOOOOOOOHHHHHH! He's so gorgeous

and soooooo BIG!' she announced, stepping from the room where the adoring couple had spent the first night of their honeymoon. 'There's only one thing wrong with Mickey, he hasn't any hair on his chest. Not a single hair. I'm a girl who's always liked hairy men.'

It was then that Jayne's IQ began to let her down and she began to have affairs with geeks of the first order. Matt Cimber was next on her list, and he beat her up constantly, but even Matt made Jayne wax lyrical at her almost daily press conferences: 'After Matt kissed me I didn't believe I'd ever been kissed before. I felt like I'd been a virgin all my life.'

At this even Matt is reported to have lifted a laconic eyebrow heavenwards.

In private she confided that she couldn't even get out of bed without Matt's permission.

In between all this activity, Jayne was having problems with her eldest daughter, Jayne Marie. She caught her youthful Latin lover Douglas with a huge hard-on in his trunks in the swimming pool with Jayne Marie, and her shriek of 'I'm SHOCKED!' echoed around the Palace. Douglas managed to make it up with the bombshell saying, 'I dreenk to you be-yoo-tee', and peace reigned temporarily.

The final straw in the IQ-of-160 theory comes with Mansfield's involvement, along with her husband Sam Brody, in black magic. Eager for another angle for their

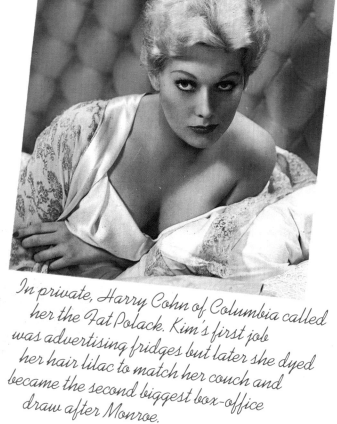

In private, Harry Cohn of Columbia called her the Fat Polack. Kim's first job was advertising fridges but later she dyed her hair lilac to match her couch and became the second biggest box-office draw after Monroe.

endless photo sessions, Jayne went to visit the San Francisco Church of Satan, where Anton Lavey claimed to be Satan's Californian correspondent. He made Jayne a high priestess and she had her photo taken prancing around like a busty Aleister Crowley. But Anton was so fucked off by Sam the Yobbo's behaviour at the church (waving horns and skulls around and laughing) that he put a curse on them both. He told them they would die in a car accident within a year. Lavey was unmoved by Jayne's pleas to remove the curse from them. Within a year the couple died in a car accident just outside New Orleans.

My mother met Jayne Mansfield just before her death, at the Cannes Film Festival. The two of them had been placed on either side of the mayor of Cannes during a screening. My dear Mama was horrified: 'Half-way through the film I realized that the Mayor just wasn't watching the film.' Looking over to see what it was had distracted him so obviously she noticed that Miss Mansfield had withdrawn her not inconsiderable appendages from her dress and was rubbing them together in a vigorous massage.

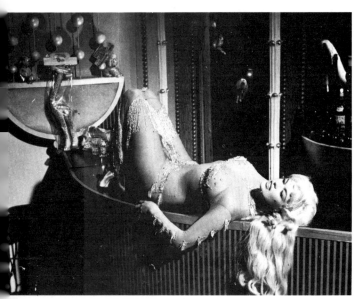

Obviously shagged from doing her Las Vegas show, the former Miss Negligée, Jayne Mansfield, relaxes on her home bar. Alongside is a gift from an admirer – a stuffed giraffe in a plastic funnel.

Jayne dieted to the point of starvation all the time in order to keep her figure in the staggering shape it maintained. She had the same measurements as Madame de Pompadour – 44–19–37, enough to make you spit.

Diana Dors

When I first arrived at the *News of the World*, where I once worked for a while, the paper was edited by a man colloquially known as 'the beast of Bouverie Street'. He was a tall thin man given to telling raucous tales of his own sex life with his wife, who was known as 'the biggest bristols in Bolton'. He was not a man with deep-rooted romance in his soul.

Nor was the rest of that office. When I first wandered into the features department I was greeted by the sounds of the features editor being harangued by a man in a raincoat shouting that he wanted three quid expenses for the job he'd just done on a cut-rate-wanking-parlour-in-Croydon. Everyone else seemed to have gone to the pub.

The subs all seemed peaceful, in their green eyeshades and hats with PRESS tickets stuck in them. In between playing poker they'd take a quick swig out of the whisky bottle in the wastepaper basket. Perhaps I exaggerate a trifle ...

But not one of them would deny the place of honour held by Diana Dors in the soaring rise to millions that the readership of this institution has enjoyed. When in America the fires were raging over Novak, Monroe and Mansfield, we in Britain enjoyed our own home-grown glamour girl. And as any self-respecting reader of the *News of the World* knows, she was one of the first women to sell her own story ...

Long before Britain was prepared to admit that all housewives outside the green belt attend 'dirty-knicker parties' and that all choirboys use preparation H, before we realized that almost the entire population except ourselves was meeting in an illicit coven behind the bicycle shed, everyone knew about Diana's torrid life.

In 1960, *News of the World* readers were thrilling to posters all over the country which gave them a taster of what was to come on Sunday. Next to a picture of a tremulous Diana (née Diana Fluck of Swindon) was the headline 'NAUGHTY GIRL'. It went on to illustrate why:

'I have a criminal record, I've been had up for house-breaking. I have modelled in scanties ... and less ... I have loved men I would rather now forget.'

You can read about the secret love life of her first husband; of the mirror on the ceiling; of the startling guest bedroom.

It's a fabulous rip-roaring life that she tells.

'I hide nothing in my story,' she says. 'I write it because I am currently a wife and about to become a mother.'

(With that intriguing non-sequitur, were we supposed to believe that Miss Dors was planning to spend her £30,000 fee on nursery equipment?)

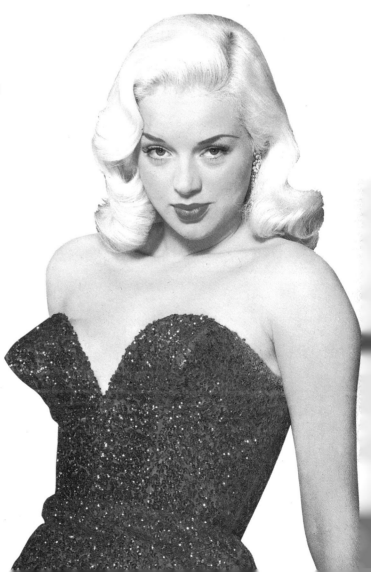

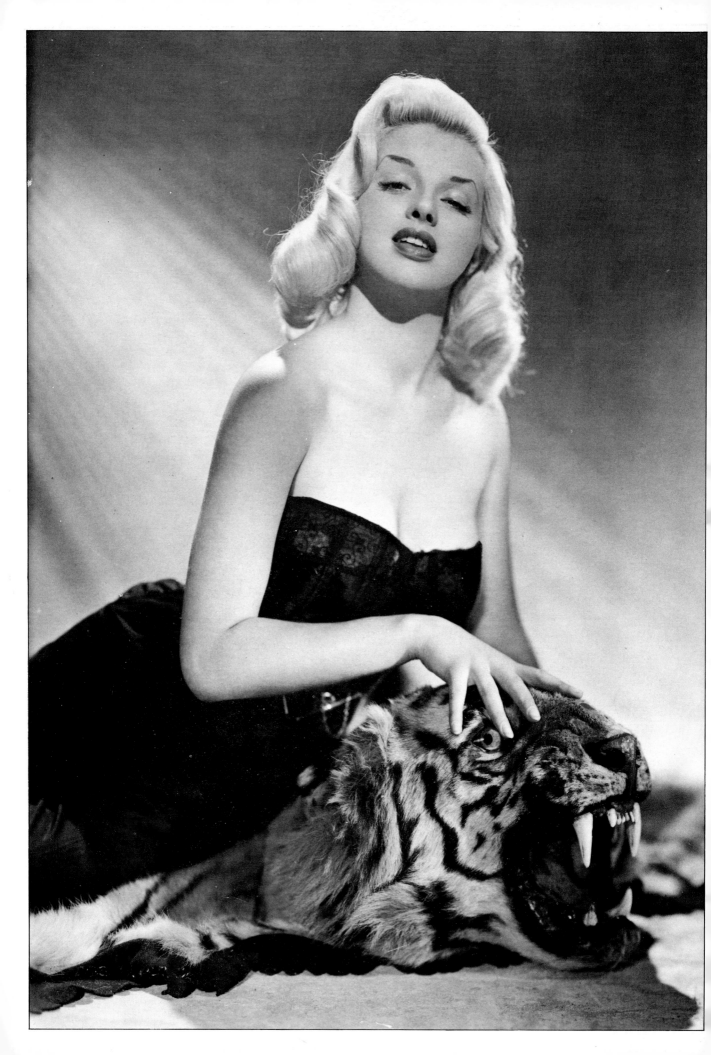

Miss Dors' tale has never been equalled, except perhaps by the *News of the World's* front-page account of a famous pop singer's paternity case, when it was alleged that he chased his quarry around a suite in Caesar's Palace squirting her with mayonnaise. Dors informed her readers that she was in the dark about her first husband's famous parties, when he used to lie on the floor looking down through the mirrored ceiling of the room below. In any case, the voyeur got the boot rapidly from Miss Dors' delicate stilleto. A few weeks later she was seen sunning herself in a mink bikini alongside actor Tommy 'Muscles' Yeardye and chewing-gum heir John Hoey.

As for the mink bikini, a truly blonde accessory if ever there was one, that was discarded after one outing.

Miss Dors later commented, while consuming a large plate of bacon and eggs in the Via Veneto, 'I have worn the mink bikini once. Where else could I wear it? I guess I'm just a recluse at heart.'

Miss Dors' other clothes lived up to the rest of her lifestyle. She sported tasteful little pink suede toreador pants with sprayed-on sequins, and her hair was a constant source of copy. Hairdresser Teasy Weasy Raymond had a special pair of 18-carat gold scissors just for cutting her hair. He was flown back and forth across the Atlantic to do her styling at a cost of about £2,500 a go. In 1956 this was considered the height of glamour, and papers never let anyone forget what an expensive head of hair she had. Among his other contributions to Western Society, Teasy also supplied the Alice band, the poodle cut, and the Teasie Weasie.

When Bob Hope asked Diana Dors to star as the girlfriend of New York Mayor Jimmy Walker, she had to say No:

It appears His Worship had an equally fabulous girlfriend, but Bob wanted me to play it. It's a great compliment for a British girl to be asked to play the part of an American glamour girl but I had to say No, mainly because they wanted me to dye my hair black. IMAGINE ME with black hair! My hair is my trade mark. It has taken me years to build up my personality and it would be silly to kill it now.

Miss Dors was taking the typically blonde stand that her hair and her personality were one and the same. Diana Dors has soared to greater and greater heights in recent years despite or perhaps because of her extra curves. In the time-honoured tradition of great blondes she possesses a black marble swimming pool, wears gold sandals and still has a staggering amount of blonde candyfloss on her head.

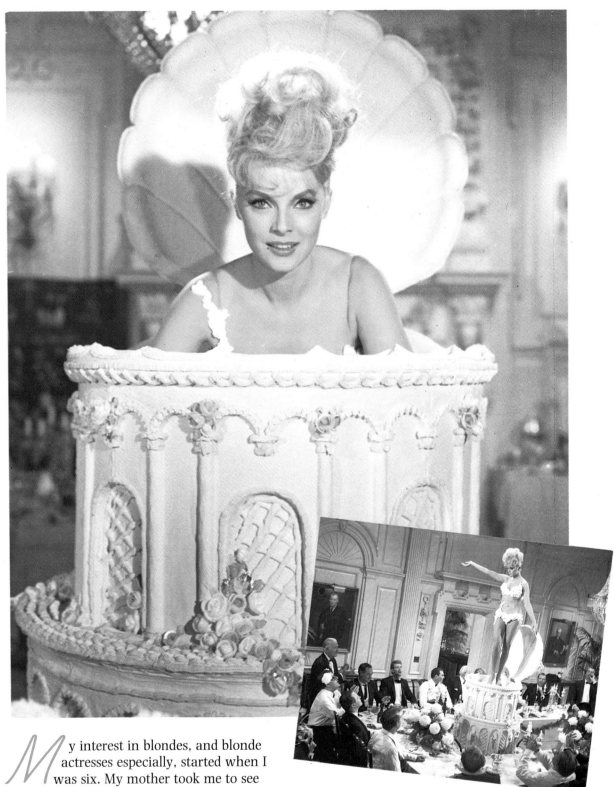

M y interest in blondes, and blonde actresses especially, started when I was six. My mother took me to see *How to Murder Your Wife*, a comedy starring Jack Lemmon and an Italian blonde called Virna Lisi. For me it was love at first sight. Not with Mr Lemmon but with Virna and her beauty spot. Virna leaped into my life out of an enormous cake, dressed in a bikini made of whipped cream. She rose out of it like the birth of Venus and I was smitten with Cupid's arrow across the Tivoli Llandudno.

Virna seemed to me, as I sat in the darkness picking a scab on my knee, a vision of loveliness. An angel. I realized that this was how everyone should look. I quickly discarded my prior ambition to grow up and be Natalie Wood. I was going to become Virna Lisi.

Several things made this rather difficult. Secretly I thought that I bore a staggering resemblance to Bruce Forsyth. My chin seemed intent on growing like something in *The Day of the Triffids*. Plus, I had hair the colour of old washing-up water. I begged my mother to let me dye my hair. She refused. I said she was unreasonable: she dyed *hers*. She lent me a wig. I wore the wig all the time until one night it was ripped off my head after I made an impromptu appearance at one of my mother's literary dinners wearing not only the wig but also her diaphragm perched jauntily on the top. 'Hello, my name's Paula what's yours,' I announced from the doorway.

After the diaphragm incident my blonde fixation cooled a little due to lack of costume. By the time I was twelve I had begun to lie on my bed reading *Cosmopolitan*. It was a magazine that dealt with important issues of the times – like whether a liberated woman should rise at dawn to put her dynel fall, false eyelashes and lip gloss on before her man woke up to see her as she really was. Sadly, as I lay there, I realized that any man taking me to bed would be waiting for me to remove my false chin.

Virna didn't have any of these soul-wrenching problems. She even had a real mole near her mouth, not a painted-on false one that smudged every time you removed your liberty bodice.

She drove around in her films in dark glasses on a pink Vespa, possessed white go-go boots like Nancy's and had toreador pants that were torrid. Whereas I appeared doomed to a life wearing my granny's double-chin strap around my face in the futile hope of making mine retreat a few feet. I had also started to kip with a peg on the end of my nose to keep it dinky, or so I thought. Estee Lauder never needed to fear my beauty tips.

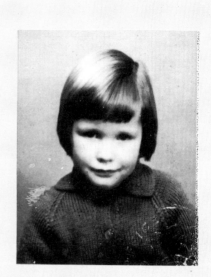

ME AGED 3

Virna's real-life existence was that of a sex kitten on the prowl. I could have puked. And she felt she owed her success to her blonde hair, having previously been a brunette in her career as an Italian starletto. George Axelrod had originally written *How to Murder Your Wife* for Marilyn. The fact that Virna barely spoke English didn't matter, we were all too busy watching her ski pants undulate like Cape Horn.

Despite language problems, Virna arrived in Hollywood custom-built for movie audience consumption. She'd already made twenty-six movies, including an atrocious toothpaste commercial where she committed a gaffe and then smiled as the announcer boomed, 'With a mouth like that she gets away with anything!' She also had a pilot's licence, half the crown jewels, thirty trunks of new Balenciagas, thirteen fur coats and seventy pairs of shoes. And three English phrases in case the going got rough: 'Is necessary?' 'Is possible' and, most improbable of all, 'Poor little Virna'.

I swooned and was allowed to dye my hair blonde when I was twelve, my mother probably desperate to nip my Forsyth look in the bud. No one could tell me that life didn't begin at twelve.

As Virna always used to say at the time, 'Always I 'ave 'ad what I wanted.'

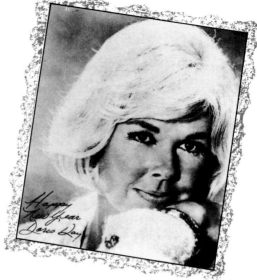

Doris Day spent most of the Sixties with a bolster down the middle of the bed trying to stave off desperate advances from a lustful Rock Hudson. From the dawn of her career as a star of frothy comedies, in *Pillow Talk* (1959), she managed to star in the same plot with a different title for eight years.

Stylish, witty, well dressed and career-minded, she was determined to keep the top half of his pyjamas on come hell or high water. Until they were both safely up the aisle.

Joe Pasternak produced her film *Jumbo* in 1962, and commented that 'she is the sort of girl that men see as someone they could spend the rest of their life with. The Elizabeth Taylor type they look upon as the sort of girl they could desire for a night. Women like her because she is the sort of woman they are themselves, they don't see her as a threat.'

Mr Pasternak was obviously carried away as he went on to wax lyrical about Doris' undoubted charms, adding, 'To the world she is the girl, not next door, but on the next lawn.'

No one ever asked what exactly he thought people visualized Miss Day doing on their lawns.

In the meantime Doris was making more light sophisticated comedies, fending off men with heads shaped like footballs. The plot was always the same: an-independent-career-woman-with-a-vast-wardrobe-being-pursued-by-a-wolf-with-a-gleam-in-his-eye.

Older audiences in particular found her a constant source of comfort during the Sixties. While Susan George was being a steamy nymphet, Julie Christie was sleeping on floors and everyone else was swinging round Chelsea, Jim Garner and Rock Hudson were still stuck with Doris and the perennial problem of Will She Or Won't She?

Her films stayed in the Top Ten from 1959 through to 1966.

Doris Day's romantic sex comedies worked because of one thing. Doris was creamy-blonde enough for you to imagine men pursuing her even if she was being utterly boring and wearing three pairs of knickers on each date, one with a pocket for a 2p in case she had to phone her mother. With Miss Day's wardrobe that was the least of their problems. In *Do Not Disturb*, a film little over an hour and a bit long, she had fifty-eight costume changes, several of which

James Garner courts Doris Day. Step-by-step guide to a hot date:

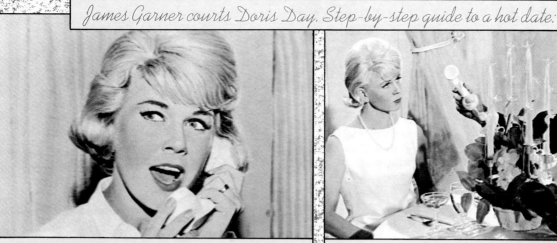

1. Doris is thrilled Jim's rung her

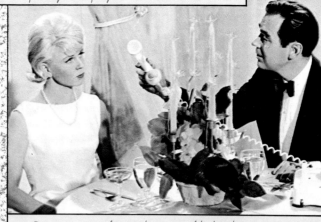

2. Dinner a deux by candlelight

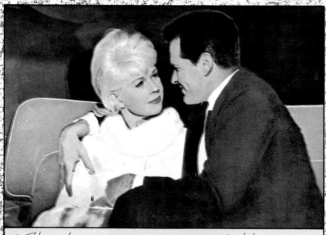

3 They kiss: a searing moment of longing

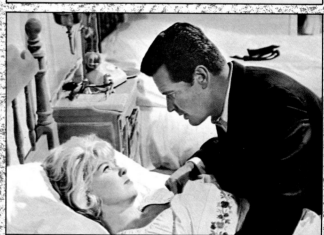

4 He gives her one

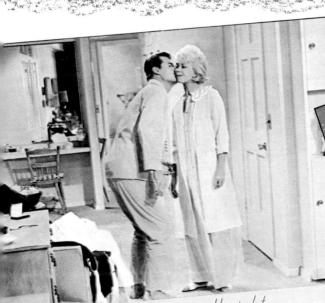

By keeping her jammies on all night,
Doris ensures that Jim'll still respect her
in the morning . . .

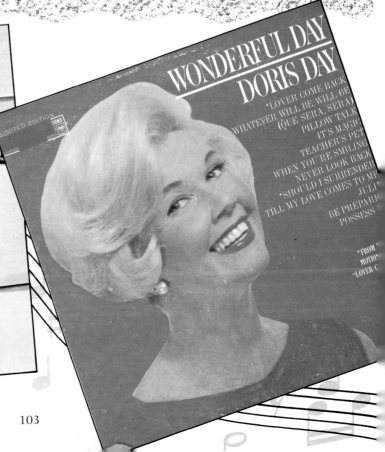

WONDERFUL DAY
DORIS DAY

*LOVER COME BACK
WHATEVER WILL BE, WILL BE
(QUE SERA, SERA)
PILLOW TALK
IT'S MAGIC
TEACHER'S PET
WHEN YOU'RE SMILING
NEVER LOOK BACK
*SHOULD I SURRENDER
TILL MY LOVE COMES TO ME
JUL
BE PREPARE
POSSESS

*FROM
MOTION
*LOVER C

LIMITED EDITION

were seen for less than twenty seconds. The clothes cost £35,700 (and that was in 1965) and shrewdly Miss Day kept the lot. So Miss Day not only had Hollywood's record for eternal virginity she also held the record for the most outfits worn by a single woman in one film.

Because she looked so clean, Doris' transformation into a steaming torch singer in *Love Me or Leave Me* was trumpeted as 'THE DAWN OF A NEW DAY'. The role had originally been intended for Ava Gardner, so that was fairly accurate. *Love Me or Leave Me* was a screen biography of the Twenties star, Ruth Etting. It was a mammoth success. *Calamity Jane*, helped by the fact that 'Secret Love' was a massive hit song, fared equally well in the box office and critically. The role of Calamity opposite Howard Keel (whose career has moved on dramatically – having had an affair with Sue Ellen he's now going at it with Miss Ellie), was PERFECT for Doris Day's terminal tomboyishness. She played a shrewish frontierswoman about to be tamed by Keel, who naturally doesn't wish to marry a girl who sticks her chewing gum under the seats.

This film, where she got to act like a yobbo and EVEN look a bit dirty, was the perfect antidote for her sweetness-and-light earlier appearances in movies like *April in Paris* and *I'll See You in My Dreams*.

Later in her career Day became disillusioned. She did The Doris Day Show on television for several seasons and then seemed to lose interest. Her love of dogs became of paramount importance to her: she started a mini dogs' home in her grounds and wore badges saying 'I LOVE DOGS' – rather a rash statement to make in Los Angeles.

Despite the hilarity caused by her eternal-virgin image, Doris Day's Sixties comedies are an art form unto themselves. Along with Nancy Sinatra in her boots, the sound of her voice and the sight of her apple-pie sweet face are immediately evocative of their time. No one can say a bad word about Doris to me. Her films proved that boys are after only one thing and her virginity is as fabled as Elizabeth I's.

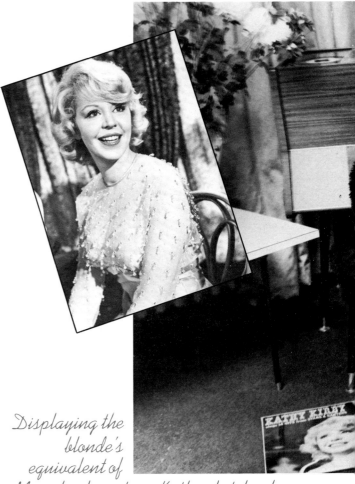

Displaying the blonde's equivalent of Memphis furniture, Kathy clutches her stuffed poodle seat.

There were those in England who imagined that, given the right breaks, Kathy Kirby might emulate Doris Day's staggering success. Unfortunately Kathy never quite made it. While almost every column inch about Day is a reference to a movie, almost every column inch about Kathy is a reference to her manager – an elderly gentleman call Bert Ambrose. One would have thought that, with a name like that, he was not a man likely to elevate a girl to the pinnacles of Hollywood stardom. Bert (or Ammie, as Kathy not surprisingly preferred to call him) had a number of ideas on how to transform his little blonde songbird.

Bert was a successful band leader of fifty-nine when he first spotted Kathy, then an unknown sixteen-year-old. Within a few

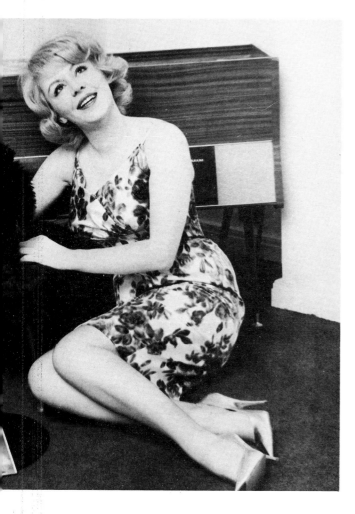

year. Then Bert thought up yet another idea to boost Kathy's image.

'I CRIED AS I WAS FORCED TO POSE TOPLESS', shrieked the headlines afterwards. Kathy claimed that Bert had become a sick and tormented man with enormous gambling debts to pay off: he'd simply decided that one way to make money was a new sultry Kathy Kirby instead of the gormless one of the past.

So there was Kathy in front of the hotlights with a blonde wig that reached her waist and NO TOP. Naturally she sobbed and ran home twisted with anguish at the thought of where she might see the pictures. Calm and collected as ever, she perched next to one of the windows and threatened to throw herself onto the pavement if Bert didn't get the negatives back immediately.

Soon after all this drama Bert died and, having been nurtured, groomed and embezzled for stardom by him, Kathy was beside herself with grief. She had become devoted to him. She also discovered how little she knew of her own affairs and each day new scandals appeared in the newspapers. The British Doris Day was lost forever.

The little girl Kathy Kirby, with her chocolate-box looks, her lisp and her crocodile patforms, was suddenly rumoured to be having a baby with Tom Jones, when she certainly wasn't. Then it was meant to be the seamy side of Pop, with drugs and drink. Finally she collapsed with a mixture of exhaustion and voice strain, probably from telling her story so many times.

Having been worth £750,000, her life was in ruins, she'd walked out on two TV series and had a row with her mother.

As she bravely struggled to keep her career afloat, Kathy Kirby's life story began to resemble a Doris Day movie. It was all beginning to sound like the Ruth Etting story, set in Bolton.

Finally Kathy decided that all she really wanted to do was get married and have children. The flags must have been put at half mast on the roof of the *News of the World* after this momentous decision. Bert robbing Kathy of her youth had filled up the papers for weeks on end.

years she was doing the Kathy Kirby Show on television, her version of 'Secret Love' sold 140,000 copies, and she went on to have hits with songs like 'Danny', 'Crush Me' and 'Now You're Crying', which were all in a sort of sexier Doris Day mould.

Bert naturally was delighted with his efforts. He took up gambling ferociously and Kathy was ensconced in a Grosvenor Square home complete with pink dralon curtains and chandeliers tinkling to the strains of her latest hits. Unfortunately for Kathy, she lacked a certain aptitude for figures and never appeared to have a clue how much she was earning. Kathy was devoted to Bert and sang 'My Yiddisher Moma' to him at the drop of a hat, which always brought tears to his eyes.

But trouble was brewing in paradise.

First Kathy went to see a palm reader who told her that Bert's days were numbered and he wasn't going to last the

Brigitte Bardot

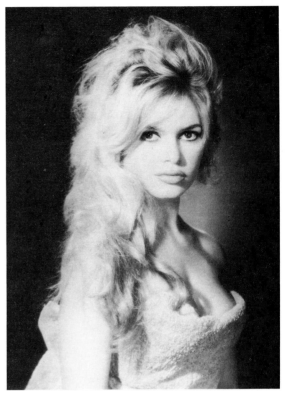

With all this blondeness across the seas, the French naturally became greatly irritated and could be found miserably flicking the ash off their Gauloises into their steaming pissoirs and moaning that France didn't have its own blonde dream girl.

Until Brigitte Bardot.

The French, despite their ill humour about almost everything, managed to come up with an almost unique blonde in this Pantheon of Famous blondes. A blonde who changed the way that people regarded the traditional glamour girl. BB became a symbol of youth, a figure of careful carelessness with tousled honey-blonde hair which tumbled down her back, and blue jeans worn with bare feet. She had none of the carefully studied artificiality of her forerunners. Bardot always looked like she'd been in bed and caused such reaction that academics started to examine her strong image. Simone de Beauvoir wrote a book about her stature as a symbol and its universal appeal.

French people, long used to traditional femme fatales, were antagonized by her and her apparent disregard for any authority. She was denounced from pulpits after her appearance in Roger Vadim's *And God Created Woman* and queues formed outside the fleapits as boys waited to examine her.

Bardot put the wank back into youth culture.

The sight of Bardot, the press coverage she received for her belief in free love ('I want no hypocrisy, no nonsense, about love'), her silly boyfriends with no brains and big muscles, her love of animals and sunbathing all contrived to make her a vision. Seeing Brigitte made one think of beaches covered in twenty-year-olds with thighs like marble, acres of topless women with sex on the brain. These were women who'd never scrubbed at their dimples with green plastic gloves filled with extract of ivy. They'd have maybe eaten the ivy. And then the glove.

Her clothes were discussed endlessly. And her lack of them. A spokeswoman for Dior commented, 'Bardot is *femme enfant*, she is not yet ready to wear our clothes, a woman's clothes.' De Beauvoir noted, 'She goes about barefoot, she turns her nose up at elegant clothes, jewels, girdles, perfumes and make-up, at all artifice.'

In reality such perfect naturalness can only be achieved after several hours of unnatural behaviour in front of a well-lit mirror, but that was beside the point.

Bardot was presented by the media as being as thoughtless as a child, sauntering through each of her film roles with an unselfconscious air. She did not appear to think deeply about anything, escept maybe her pets. As critic Pauline Kael commented, 'Bardot is the distillation of all those irresponsible petulant teenagers who may never know that human experience has a depth and expressiveness and potentialities beyond their immediate range of impulses.'

But at the end of the Fifties and the beginning of the Swinging Sixties, WHO WANTED DEPTH?

The Me-iow Generation

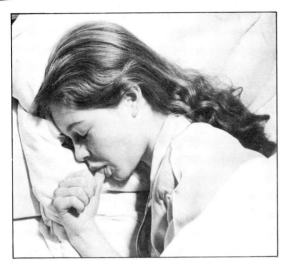

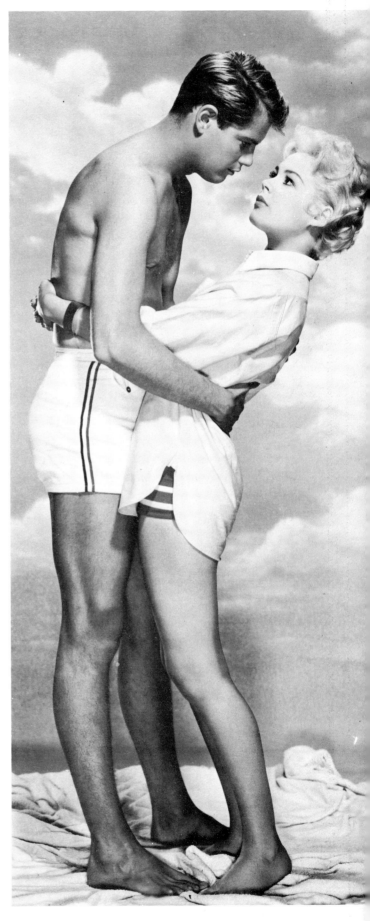

At the start of the Sixties, film makers were determined to tap a new fountain of eternal youth which had been switched on by Caroll Baker in *Baby Doll* in 1956. A stream of nubile skinny blonde actresses emerged, led by Baker, eager to put anything within a ten-mile radius into their mouths. Apart from their oral fixations, the swinging actresses of the Sixties had much else in common with their four-year-old counterparts.

Since censorship still had a strong grip on film makers, everything except the most obvious was stuffed into mouths. Sue Lyon starring as *Lolita* made a four-course meal out of one ice lolly; Sandra Dee sucked milkshake straws as though her life depended on it; and Caroll Baker and Brigitte Bardot had thumbs like raw liver after a hard day on set in their cots.

Winceyette pyjamas for the first time became *de rigueur* for the blossoming sex kitten, along with baby dolls and ankle socks.

Rather than seeing it as something threatening, as teenage movies at the end of the Fifties had become, the Sixties turned teenage frustration into a well-stuffed wild bikini doing the frug on a beach. Natalie Wood no longer died of frustration over Warren Beatty, Marlon had nothing to rebel about and Dean had died. Far from the days when Montgomery Clift, Brando and Dean had made the shortsighted watery squint a prerequisite of male sexuality, the early

Sixties boys were big blonde and dumb. The Tab Hunters and Troy Donahues of this world were never the sort of boys who threatened to pee on your leather jacket in tribal gangland initiation rites.

The teenage market was being done for every dollar it could spend. Movies catered to audiences wanting to see nice clean teenagers involved in an eternal courtship dance over a Bar-B-Que on the beach. Any time these time-honoured rituals of Californian teenage life looked like they were getting steamy, waves would crash, strings would grow lush and the screen would transmogrify into a glorious sunset like piles.

Trying to imagine Troy and Sandra Dee in the throes of coitus is like trying to visualize Isla Saint Clair nude. They seemed capable of enjoying their gilded youth without any carnal desires rearing their ugly heads. Troy was such a wet in those days that audiences felt tempted to cheer when he managed a sentence of more than six syllables. His shorts held no promise of things to come by the camp fire. Camp rather than fire was inevitably the operative word with Troy. Troy was the sort of boy who still stirred his tea with it, and for that very reason unlikely to scare you out of your wits at the drive-in.

He was the perfect boyfriend for any teenage girl.

Despite Troy's lack of passions and Sandra's desire to nab her man almost to the exclusion of any other activity, these teenage beach movies are the nearest that Americans have ever got to capturing the essence of languid drifting summers, the sort you never enjoy again after the age of fifteen. But sadly Americans find this ideal totally against their natures. How can you enjoy a gilded languid youth if you're worrying about your acne and your braces?

Sandra Dee had the misfortune to have to play a character whose name was a composite of Girl and Midget and then, even worse, to be typecast in the role. The films were incredibly popular and put Dee into the Top Ten of box office stars for the early part of the decade. In each, as Sandra wriggled off to the beach in her shorts, her mother was there at the gingham-upholstered kitchen door to remind her that the family motto was, 'To be a real woman is to bring out the best in a man', or some such sentiment.

Natalie Wood would have shuddered in the grass.

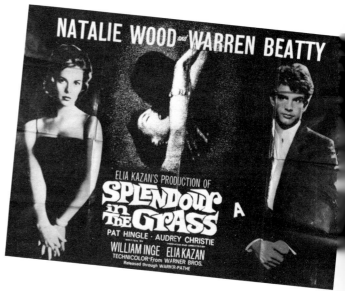

After a couple of films together, the blood finally found its way from Troy's ears to his loins and naturally Sandra got knocked up first time. Sandra Dee? *In trouble?* the nation was on tenterhooks in the odeons. Never before had Troy and Sandra had to deal with such an adult problem and they did it with aplomb and plenty of singing in the background from a thousand-voice choir from the Mormon Tabernacle. Never before had so much hedging of the broader issues had to be done in one film.

A Summer Place was a smash. The sexy theme which heralded all the smutty moments went to number one in the charts and became the song to get laid to in 1963.

James Dean was proof that you don't need good eyesight or a small behind in order to become a blonde legend.

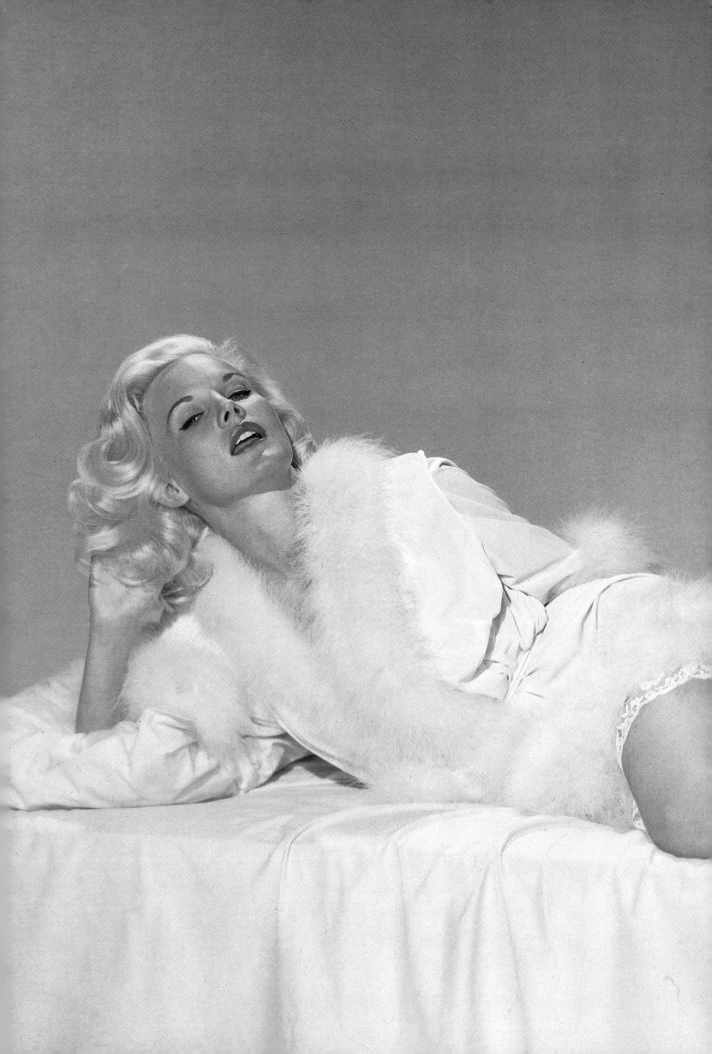

Carroll Baker

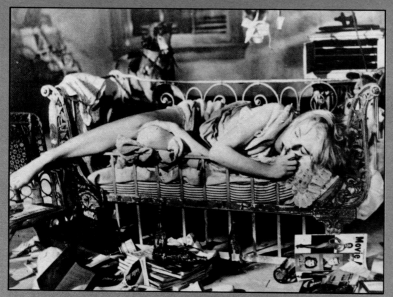

Baby Doll was so sultry even the walls sweated.

In her *tour de force* as Karl Malden's adulterous child-bride, she stole away some of the steam that until then had been the sole preserve of Elizabeth Taylor in a slip and Paul Newman in his vest. Carroll was never like all the other teenagers looking like scalded hams on the beach, she was steaming in the kitchen in dirty pjs with sweat trickling off her blonde hair like it was melting.

Carroll Baker had become everyone's dream baby in *Baby Doll* back in '56, but she retained her crown as Queen of the Thumbsuckers well into the Sixties.

She was the doyenne of repressed, steaming teenage sexuality. She was the girl that Tenessee Williams must have dreamed of. No one ever recovered from the sight of Baker in a filthy cot surrounded by gossip magazines.

Despite this momentous moment in screen sex, where every man was suddenly able to admit he longed for an overgrown school girl in a cot in the spare bedroom, Miss Baker's career took a nose dive. Curiously she found herself in the odd position of being a serious actress who took the easy way out by making sexy films. Normally it was the sex symbols who dreamed of being taken seriously.

She appeared in *Station Six Sahara* as the

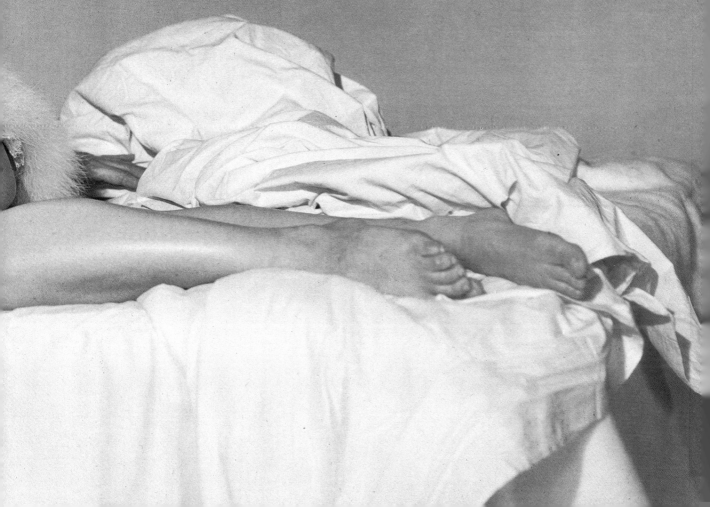

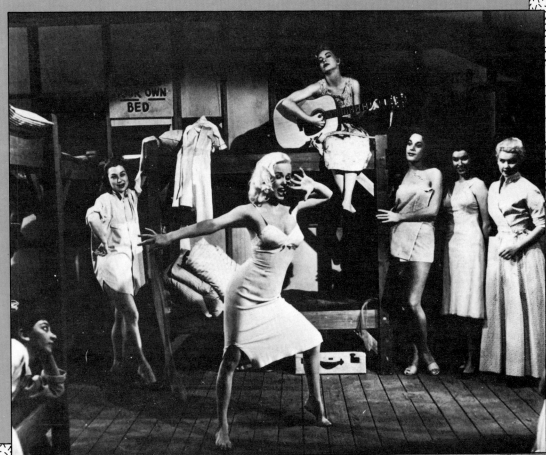

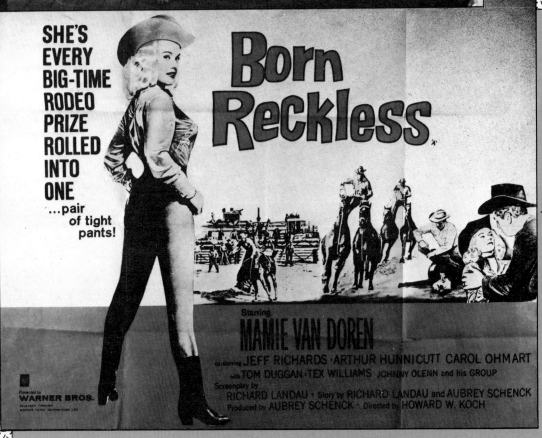

SHE'S
EVERY
BIG-TIME
RODEO
PRIZE
ROLLED
INTO
ONE
...pair
of tight
pants!

Born Reckless

Starring
MAMIE VAN DOREN

co-starring JEFF RICHARDS · ARTHUR HUNNICUTT · CAROL OHMART
with TOM DUGGAN · TEX WILLIAMS · JOHNNY OLENN and his GROUP
Screenplay by
RICHARD LANDAU · Story by RICHARD LANDAU and AUBREY SCHENCK
Produced by AUBREY SCHENCK · Directed by HOWARD W. KOCH

Presented by
WARNER BROS.
RELEASED THROUGH
WARNER-PATHÉ DISTRIBUTORS LTD

lone woman driving six men insane with desire. Most of the press wasn't about her acting, it was all about her Pierre Balmain wardrobe which she sensibly arranged to keep after the film was over. She even got the ermine coat, worth £3,500. (Worried that, when she was stabbed in the film, the coat might be ruined, Pierre inserted a little piece of white rabbit fur in the back.) She was also togged up with a gown called Rose de Paris, trimmed all over with roses, and a pink cocktail dress trimmed with diamonds and pink straw tufts. When asked by bemused press-men whether all this wasn't a trifle extreme for a film about throbbing thighs in the desert, she replied 'Nah, they dress for dinner.'

At twenty-nine she still looked twelve and not everything was running smoothly. In the middle of her passionate love scene on Broadway with Van Johnson, a little man in the front row leaped up and threw a bit of paper at her. It was a writ demanding £23,680 from Warners. Afterwards a shocked and stunned Miss Baker complained, 'That was the most dastardly thing that anybody could do to an actress in the middle of a performance.'

She then went off to find fame, fortune and family in Italy.

Mamie van Doren

While all of this activity was going on, Mamie Van Doren was starring in some of the greatest titles of the twentieth century. Dire dross the films may have been, but the titles were enough to seduce any movie goer. During her career Mamie brought her own unique brand of Method Acting to films like *Born Reckless, The Girl in Black Stockings, High School Confidential, Beat Generation, Sex Kittens Go to College, The Private Lives of Adam and Eve, The Navy Versus The Night Monsters* and finally *Voyage to the Planet of the Prehistoric Women*.

With names like that the directors obviously felt plots could be dispensed with.

Mamie often acted like Mr Ed the Talking

Horse and some say she was the forerunner of the Farrah Fawcett school of acting. With an important line like, 'Over yonder', Mamie could make a seven-minute scene just licking her lips and pointing in the wrong direction.

Acting alongside Mamie in *Sex Kittens Go to College* was Tuesday Weld. Christened Susan, she became a child model called Tu Tu, which then changed to Tuesday. She appeared in a number of films with plots like Sandra Dee's and titles like *Rock Rock Rock*. Then she was in *Return to Peyton Place* as the girl who kills the man who's raped her, and in *Wild in the Country* (with Elvis Presley) as an unmarried guitar-strumming mother.

Tuesday Weld became a serious actress later in her career after these early epics. According to George Axelrod, 'Tuesday's a great actress because she doesn't fake anything and the reason she doesn't fake anything is because she can't.'

After her marriage to Roddy McDowell's secretary she turned down some good parts. Among the films that Tuesday didn't do after the birth of her baby were *Cactus Flower, True Grit* and *Bonnie and Clyde*.

But then that's the kind of thing you do if you're a wild untamed youth whose heart belong to Waikiki.

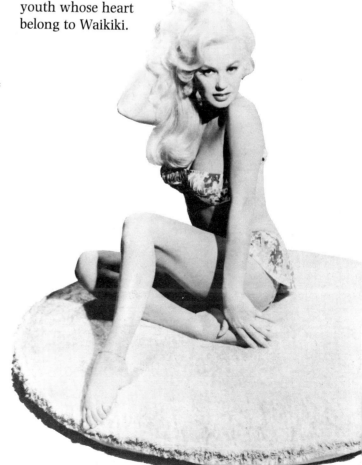

If I've one life to live, let me live it as a Blonde

Possibly the blonde's finest moment during the Sixties was when Nancy Sinatra swung along the cat walk at 'Top of the Pops' wearing a white mini dress, a Swahili suntan and those memorable mid-calf white plastic boots. Shaking the contents of her mini dress she mimed those immortal words, shook her long blonde hair and everyone realized that this was an easy time to be a blonde.

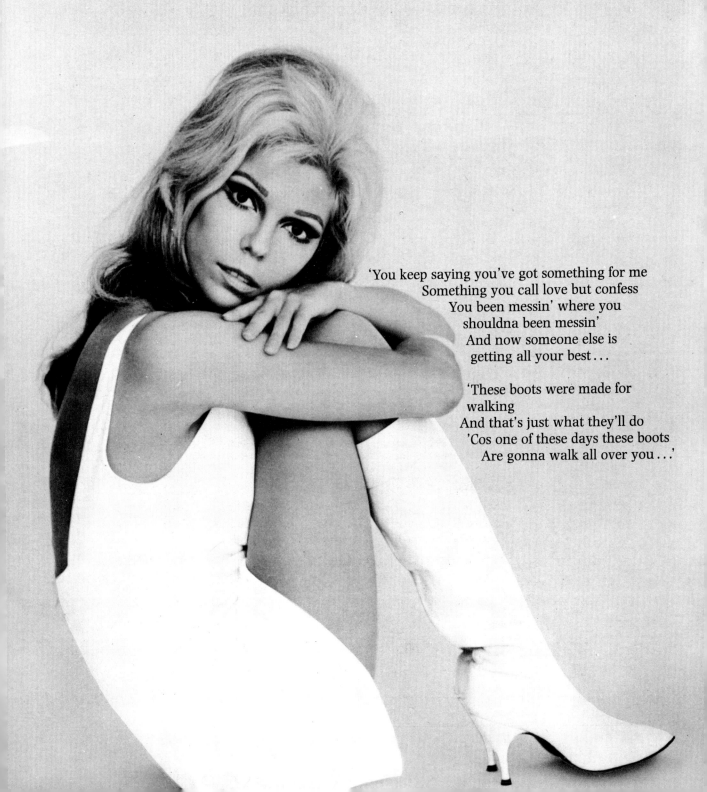

'You keep saying you've got something for me
Something you call love but confess
You been messin' where you
shouldna been messin'
And now someone else is
getting all your best . . .

'These boots were made for
walking
And that's just what they'll do
'Cos one of these days these boots
Are gonna walk all over you . . .'

During the Sixties it suddenly became incredibly easy to dye one's hair. And the range of colours that the home dyer could use was phenomenal. As she sat on the loo with a plastic bag on her head, the would-be blonde could either become a White Minx, a Frivolous Fawn, get a Chocolate Kiss or even be Tickled Pink, all courtesy of Clairol. Life took on whole new colours in 1963.

One French firm boasted 254 colours and by 1968 in Britain twenty nationally advertised dye companies were sharing an annual turnover of £9 million.

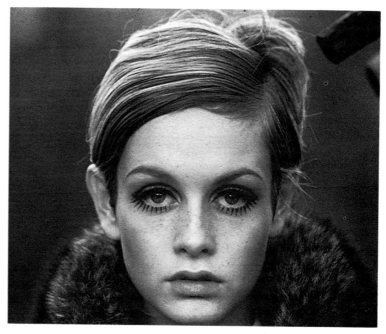

The great question – what do people DO for fun in countries where there are no blondes? – was finally answered. They still dye their hair but it goes a funny red colour if they're not careful. The Japanese became one of Clairol's biggest markets and have maintained that position ever since.

Even China fell for the blonde. After years of almost electrocuting themselves in order to get perms, and all the horrors of the Cultural Revolution when plaits were chopped off in the street and anything other than a simple pudding-basin style was deemed a symbol of the bourgeoisie and therefore illegal, suddenly Chinese girls wanted to be reborn blonde.

In London the streets were filled with women making every effort to look eleven, with fair hair, whimsical clothes and dope

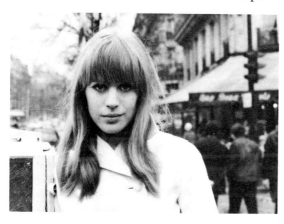

growing in their bathrooms. Twiggy, considered universally as The Face and The Blonde of the Decade, was considered the gauche epitome of ideal coltishness. Pop stars put their seal of approval on all this gilded youth: Brian Jones wandered around with Anita Pallenberg, Mick starred in *Performance* with the gloriously blonde James Fox and stepped out with Marianne Faithful. The dreadful Twinkle wore three inches of make-up and sang about her boyfriend Terry driving into a tree. Dusty Springfield was the leading antipodean blonde, later followed by Olivia Newton John. And then there were the really triff blondes who had Mary Quant white go-go boots with built-in see-through heels, mini skirts three inches wide and Mr Freedom jumpers with fried eggs on the front.

The Sixties made it easy to be blonde. The famous copy line by Shirley Polykoff, 'If I only have one life to live – Let me live it as a blonde', was like a chant in hairdressing salons.

The actresses of the Sixties conformed to the general ideal of looking eleven. Twiggy jetted off to the States to answer important questions like, 'Why are you so skinny?', and psychologists felt it had got to the point where they should say something.

In 1969, an eminent shrink commented: 'If a man is serious about a girl, he wants

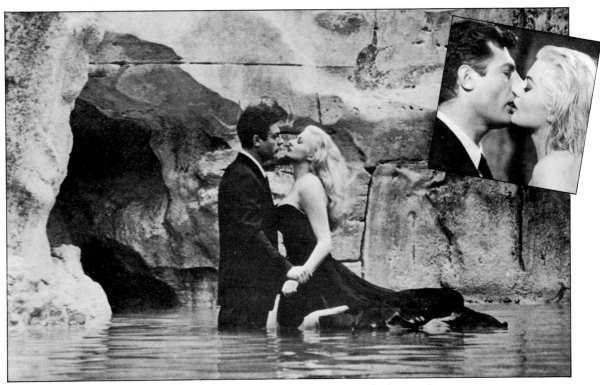

Practising for New Year's Eve at Trafalgar Square?

her to be natural. Anything artificial does not appeal to a serious-thinking man who values quality.' But none of these lithe free spirits appeared to know any serious-thinking men, he continued later in a national paper. 'Generally speaking, a man prefers a blonde for a mistress and a brunette for a wife.'

I was too young at this stage to have ANY FUN. The only treats I got were watching the reasonably blonde Dr Kildare for whom I harboured a mad crush. My week was made up of waiting for Dr Kildare and then sitting only inches from the screen for the opening credits. These showed Dr Kildare at work, occasionally pausing for a freeze frame of him and his ever-active stethoscope.

During the freeze frames I would attach my lips to the screen like a ravenous squid, only to let go of whatever bit of his anatomy I hit when the credits rolled again.

The rest of the week was spent recovering from these fleeting moments of sin with the unknowing Richard Chamberlain.

My older friends had moved on from this sort of juvenile behaviour and were watching 'Peyton Place' in groups. 'Peyton Place' had to be watched in groups because then you could pool your knowledge of sex and follow what was going on in the plot. 'Peyton Place' was a breeding ground for WASP Americans with Mia Farrow, Ryan O'Neal and Lana Turner stabbing and kissing their way through the cast. Mia the blonde urchin was a favourite with the press. When she began her affair with Frank Sinatra the papers almost pulped themselves with the excitement, which was only matched when she chopped off her long blonde hair in a fit of pique with Frankiepoo.

Sex hadn't hit TV in the Sixties. 'I Dream of Jeannie', with Barbara Eden in harem pants, was the nearest it got . . . we had to wait for Farrah and her crew for that.

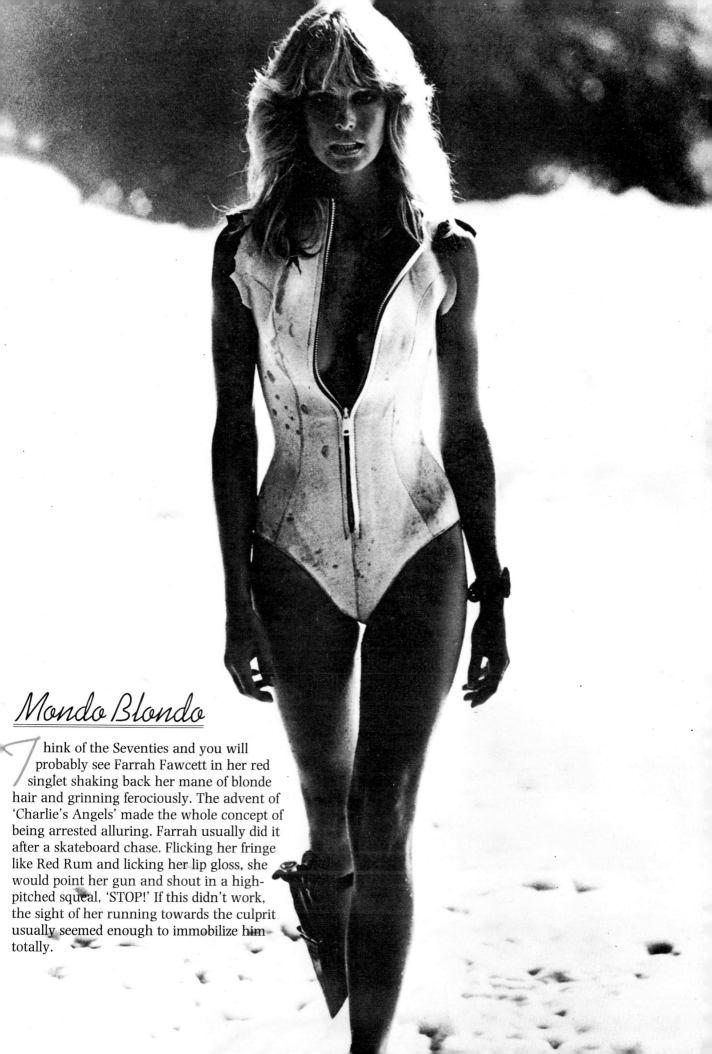

Mondo Blondo

Think of the Seventies and you will probably see Farrah Fawcett in her red singlet shaking back her mane of blonde hair and grinning ferociously. The advent of 'Charlie's Angels' made the whole concept of being arrested alluring. Farrah usually did it after a skateboard chase. Flicking her fringe like Red Rum and licking her lip gloss, she would point her gun and shout in a high-pitched squeal, 'STOP!' If this didn't work, the sight of her running towards the culprit usually seemed enough to immobilize him totally.

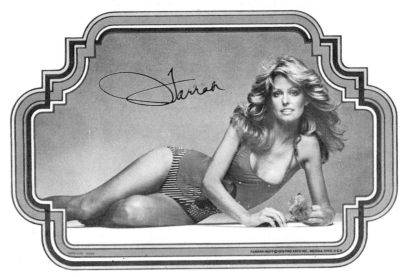

Farrah was followed by Cheryl Ladd, and the stars of soap operas like 'Flamingo Road' (which boasted a bitchy blonde called Morgan Fairchild who appeared to have every single article of clothing trimmed with maribou feathers) and 'Dallas' – which soared to the top of the ratings with Pam the brunette who says, 'Geeve me taime, Bob-bee,' at the start of every kiss; the poison dwarf, a blonde with almost no neck or legs who was cruelly cast as a woman who loves to wear shorts; Afton, a blonde who bursts into song and has runny eyes all the time; and several others, including one called Donna who's the token intelligent woman and naturally not quite as pretty as the rest of the cast.

But at least she doesn't have to stand on a box in order to kiss anything more than a zipper.

'Dynasty', 'Dallas'' nearest rival, had one of John Derek's ex-wives Linda Evans as the icily beautiful Krystle. Like Bo and Ursula, Linda appears to have been carved out of marble. She also has a permanent look of relief on her face, probably because she's not having to endure Mr Derek snatching toffees out of her mouth in public like he does with Bo.

The advent of glam rock brought fatal androgyny into the early Seventies, with groups like the Sweet, men like Bowie and various other dyed blonde bombshells who turned out to be boys, like David Johansen in the New York Dolls with their ripped girls' blouses and red ankle socks, and Iggy Pop with his dodgy hairstyle and odd habits.

Even Dolly Parton admitted she wore a wig and a specially constructed corset to hold everything up and in. Questions Questions Questions . . . you could never be sure in the Seventies what you were getting.

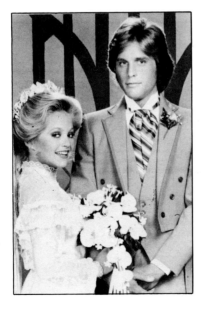

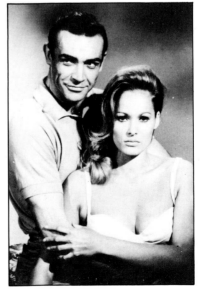

There was one star though with whom one could have some certainty. Debbie Harry in *Blondie* captured all the fun and cartoonish sexuality of her comic-strip counterparts like Augusta, Jane and the real Blondie. Wriggling and pouting in micro-minis and a lion's mane of fake blonde hair, she set schoolboys back months in their O level swotting and brought a fresh lease of life to girl singers who longed to bring back the Nancy Sinatra style of song.

Apart from the odd exceptions, in the Seventies the best thing to be apart from blonde was a boy.

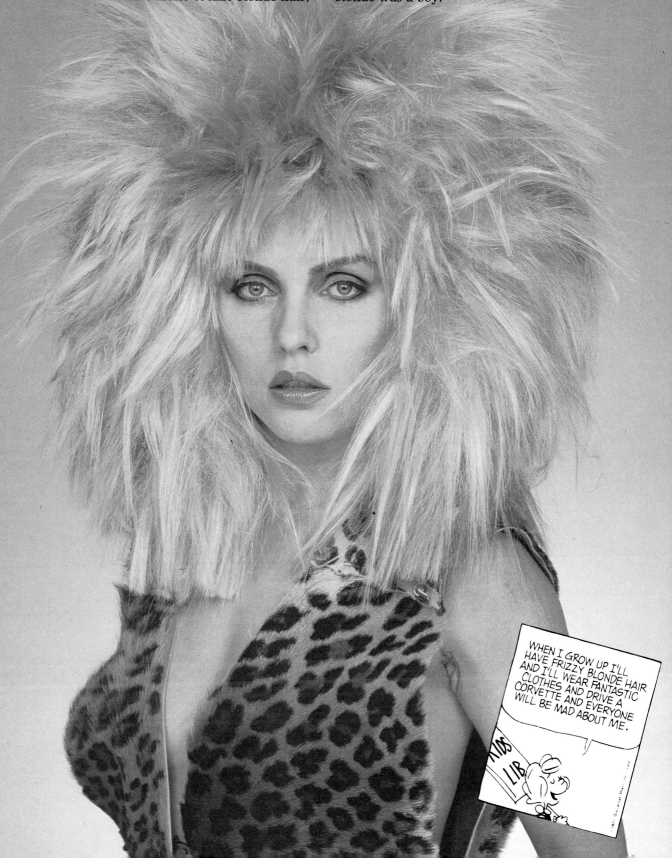

WHEN I GROW UP I'LL HAVE FRIZZY BLONDE HAIR AND I'LL WEAR FANTASTIC CLOTHES AND DRIVE A CORVETTE AND EVERYONE WILL BE MAD ABOUT ME.

KIDS LIB

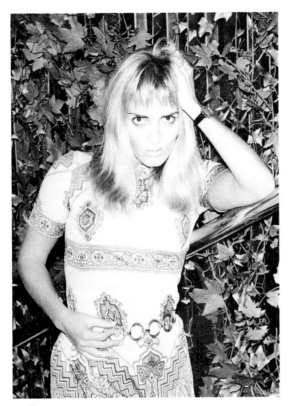

'I'm making more money vertically than I used to make horizontally,' said Xaviera gleefully when her novel *The Happy Hooker* became a bestseller. 'Anyway, after 3,000 I lost count of the number of men I've made love to,' she added, in case we be in any doubt as to her abilities.

The book described in fairly graphic terms Miss Hollander's rise to the top of her profession, so to speak.

But because of her fame as a madam, her other exploits also received massive publicity. She stole three nighties and hit the headlines, probably because no one could imagine what this woman was going to do with three winceyette nighties unless she was planning to use them as ropes. She made an album of groaning noises, interspersed with tales of fucking the man who came to fix the Potterton boiler and 'how I got the burn mark off the Wilton carpet as he dragged me rampantly from room to room'. It was also available on tapes, a fact which worried the AA so much that they advised British drivers not to play it while moving in case of accidents. A piece of advice that could have been taken all manner of ways. Naturally worried about their customers' safety, Timothy Whites banned the offending tapes.

Xaviera, if one listened to her outpourings, had been mixing with the right sort of boys. 'Spanking is a very widespread (!) sex practice in England,' she informed everyone, going on to describe a weekend party she'd attended, 'when I got my first lesson in what the aristocracy does for kicks . . . The house was thick with Lords.'

Had she had any real knowledge of the British upper classes, Xaviera would have realized immediately that she had been accidentally invited to the Old Boys Reunion. In between discussing Catholic dogma, 'Does Angst have a place in O Levels?' and whether it was right that they should have spent their entire youth arranging kissing races in the swimming pool and wearing their trunks in the showers, these men 'all talked of their school days where a matron or a master, a surrogate nanny, one said, used to beat them'.

Xaviera was baffled but keen, so after three Hail Marys and a couple of Stations of the Cross she set to work. 'This was my most lasting impression of the aristocracy – their desire to get spanked.'

It is obvious in retrospect that Xaviera missed her true calling and should have been a researcher for *Burke's Peerage*.

Fiona Richmond was a simple Norfolk vicar's daughter until she discovered her rare and often stunning talent for thinking of odd sexual positions and situations. And then writing them all down with her cheeks still firmly sucked in.

She can safely claim to be one of the few erotic writers to have included scenes such as heroines who get given one through the holes in a hammock by a wild and desperate lover who has positioned himself underneath with his willie waving seductively in the air. She can also claim to be one of the few writers to have written athletic erotic passages involving all manner of accoutrements without the air being expelled from her carefully-sucked-in cheeks with a loud farting noise.

Fiona Richmond is the sort of woman who's found her G spot. In fact the whole tale of the G spot sounds like one of Fiona's plots. 'Nurse Whipple was working in the lab with a doctor Graffenburg when she decided in the interests of science to stick her finger up his bum, etc. etc. . . .'

WHAT KIND OF AN OFFICE WAS THIS? If I were to wander nonchalantly across *Cosmopolitan*'s g-plan offices and stick my finger up the chief sub's backside, the screams would be heard in Woking. However, Nurse Whipple got away with it and the two of them discovered her G spot.

It could easily have come from Miss Richmond's biro. With bestselling books blessed with titles like *Throb*, and a twelve-foot mirror in her bedroom reflecting not some massive Ken Norton figure brandishing a candle, but the spires and sportsgrounds of Winchester Cathedral and College, she is living proof that a fertile imagination and a way with words can pay.

She has also packed them in from Torquay to Torbay in thespian epics like *Wot No Pyjamas* and *Space in My Pyjamas*. Despite their titles these comedies virtually never saw a pyjama. Although Miss Richmond did once get pelted with coins by a rowdy mob of students attending *Wot No Pyjamas*, no one seemed to object at all.

My only contact with Miss Richmond ended with me and a fellow journalist sitting like rouge-faced schoolgirls in the front row of a TV chat show on which all three of us were about to devastate the country with our wit on the topic of humour.

Miss Richmond's dress plunged like a kingfisher spotting a fat sardine in a freezing river and she spent almost the entire first fifteen minutes of the programme sucking her face in, pressing her bosoms

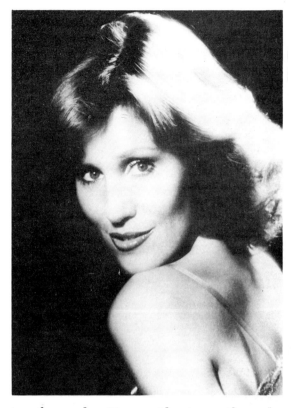

together and writing rapid notes on the pad in front of her. Naturally Miss Henessy and I (total bust-size approximately 29 inches) were gripped by the green-eyed monster. This vast expanse of CLEAVAGE was obviously either clamped together with surgical sutures or held in place with gaffer tape. It couldn't be real, we muttered tetchily.

HA! the notes she was writing while everyone else chatted on, they were obviously her next three books.

'His hot breath pounded against her thighs,' I whispered.

'Her hand rested upon his iron tool,' said Val.

'She groaned, "Your body's like a spanner . . . It tightens my nuts",' quoth I.

This merry interchange between me and Val was sadly brought to an end during the commercial break when the producer of the show rather sheepishly approached us both and mentioned that due to the odd acoustics in the studio Miss Richmond was able to hear everything we were saying and was finding it most disconcerting.

My days as a porn writer ended under her piercing glare for the next half hour.

Eat your heart out, Mark Spitz.

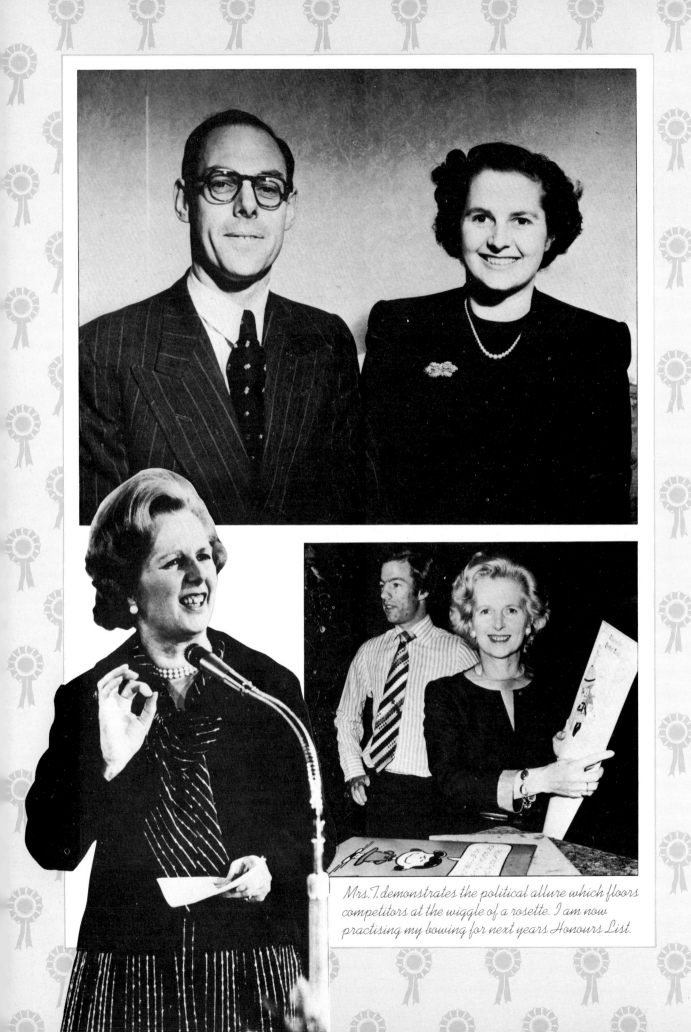

Mrs. T. demonstrates the political allure which floors competitors at the wiggle of a rosette. I am now practising my bowing for next years Honours List.

Great Blonde Conservatives

*T*estimonials to Mrs Thatcher's potent allure are not hard to come by.

According to Norman Mailer, who was covering the 1983 General Election, Mrs T. looked 'scrumptious enough to kiss'. Mr Mailer – a man with eight children, a massive chest and a bionic biro – had obviously been astonished by this sudden grasp on the secret of Mrs Thatcher's appeal.

Her husband Denis says that when he first gazed at her across a crowded Conservative Association meeting, 'She was beautiful, gay, very kind and thoughtful. This is, of course, her greatest quality. Who could meet Margaret without being completely slain by her personality and intellectual brilliance.'

Even foreigners cannot remain untouched by this secret *femme fatale* of Conservatism. One enraptured Arab admirer wrote an ode to her which was later published in national newspapers.

It is clear from all this devotion that one must look at Mrs Thatcher with new eyes. Even though Mrs T. may have said, 'I don't think there are any advantages to being a woman, if you are the premier', there obviously are. As elections and budgets approach, Mrs T's hair becomes paler, and

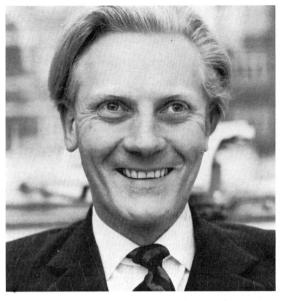

her press photos are suddenly shot through a pair of tights. On her trip to China she must have taken particular care of her coiffure: when she tripped up, the commentator was only worried she might 'break her hair'. Now, with success surrounding her, her hair rises like Vesuvius erupting on top of her head.

Mrs Thatcher is becoming positively honey blonde.

Following her lead, so is Michael Heseltine, who obviously feels that if Crumpetism works for Maggie it'll work for him. He's photographed with his arms flexed above his straight blonde flick, relaxing on trains. Michael is the opposite sort of blonde to Mrs T. Nicknamed Tarzan, he adopts the casual blonde style, his blue shirts rolled a little, his wrist-watch casually turned inwards. Heseltine is naturally the darling of the Conservative Party Conferences – not just because of his talents as an orator, but also because he's something nice to look at after all those fat boys with big rosettes coming in on behalf of the Young Tories.

Not since the Kennedys has sex put votes in the ballot boxes so successfully. Mrs Thatcher makes the veins pulse in men's temples, one only has to look at Arthur Scargill (another blonde, or at least what's left of it) to see veins pulsing in his temples at the thought of her.

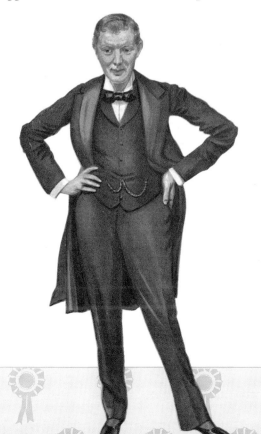

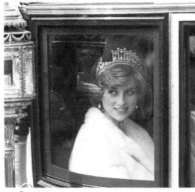
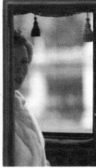

*J*ust as politicians seem to fare better with blonde hair, the same applies to Princesses. From fairy stories to real life the perfect Princess is eternally fair. Ever since Princess Diana first ventured shyly out of Coleherne Court completely upholstered in Laura Ashley her streaks have got steadily wider and wider until now there're no brown bits in between.

Well on the way to becoming the first platinum Princess of Wales, she's been on every cover there is.

Her first coup was to get photographed at her kindergarten surrounded by angelic children, with a beam of light shining straight through her skirt and NO SLIP IN EVIDENCE.

The reaction was as if she'd been caught wearing a corset and red suspenders. Her only comment was a wry one about her legs being like a piano's, which made everyone adore her even more ... even Charles must have started to realize that, although the Press were making her look hunted, she appeared to be using all the tactics of a golden Botticelli-faced Rommel with her flat-mates acting as desert rats.

Since the days of swotting for her raffia-work O Level, Lady Diana had had a sneaking regard for Charles and had even kept a photo of him by her bed, as it was later reported by a super-grass from her boarding school to the fact-hungry tabloids. They had met when she was still a baby and the affair seemed to have been created by angels in heaven.

The romance it seems was cemented when the couple met in a muddy field.

Blushing, wellington-clad and wearing her husky no doubt, Diana was probably wishing she had that corset with red suspenders on when she saw Charles across the crowded field.

He thought she was 'fraffly jolly'.

I sighed almost continuously throughout the whole romance along with everyone else in the world.

The only teensy uncomfortable moments were when her family, who have always had close ties with the Royal Family, started declaring her virginity like some tribe from Senegal. The Brits shifted in their armchairs a trifle worried that Charles was going to wave the blood-stained sheets over the balcony of Buck House. We all knew that Diana was a Princess down to her toes and I was quite willing to believe that, put to the test, she had the sort of Royal Bottom that could feel peas through twenty-two mattresses.

It is a little-known fact (among the many I've made up in this vast and varied book of history) that I attended the Royal Wedding. A newspaper impressed by my intense patriotism sent me and I sat within gobbing distance of the Queen and Randy Andy and within glaring distance of the pile of diamonds on Raine Spencer's right shoulder.

I started howling at the arrival of the bride. By the time Kiri te Kanawa was giving it all she'd got, looking like a sherbet dip on a hot night, I had two lumps of tissue paper inserted rather unglamorously into each nostril, donated kindly by the *New Zealand Times* correspondent who'd worn a morning suit. 'I Vow to Thee My Country', a tune of particular significance to me, sent me into a paroxysm of weeping due to an excess of feeling proud to be British and so close to Prince Andrew and his teeth.

Back home with the TV I sobbed afresh at the glories of the dress, the glories of the flower arrangements which I hadn't been able to see at the time because of a badly placed pillar in St Paul's and the trumpet playing.

My granny rang me up and was playing her cornet down the phone to celebrate the

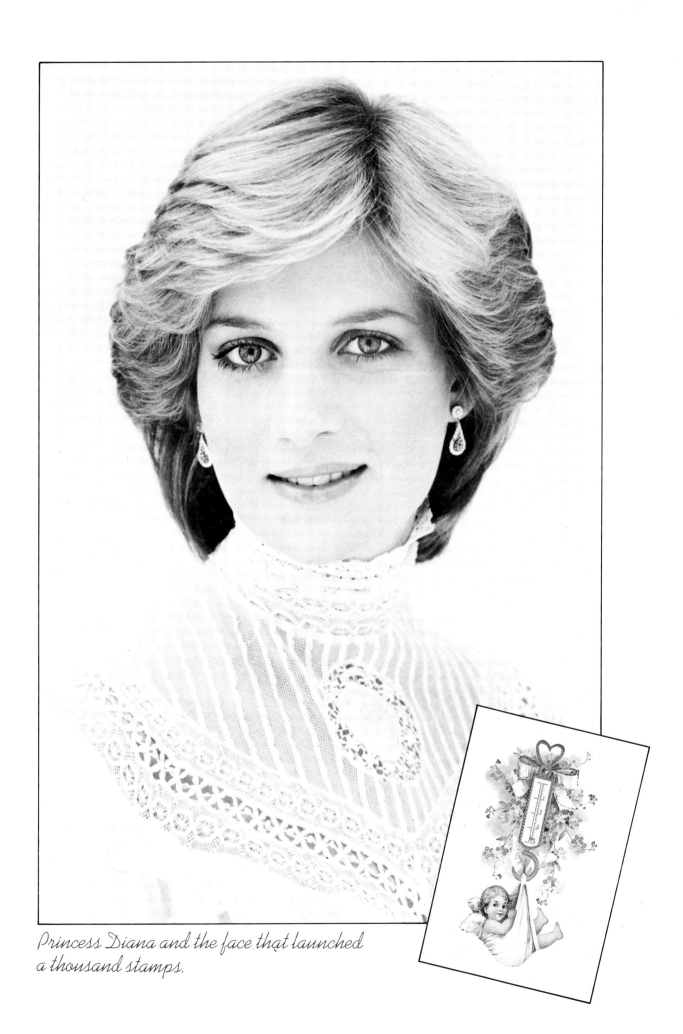

*Princess Diana and the face that launched
a thousand stamps.*

whole occasion when both of us were stunned into a temporary silence by the sudden appearance of the bride's step-grandmother Barbara Cartland, dressed as Rosa Kleb in a St John's Ambulance uniform, giving her message of romance on the news. For some mysterious reason, room had not been found for Miss Cartland at the Ceremony, possibly in case she whipped up in a little number that upstaged the bride.

As for the dress, Britain should be grateful that Diana's wedding dress didn't throw them into quite such a frenzy as the black dress the Emmanuels designed for her first official engagement. After she'd bunny-dipped out of the limousine in that bold black ballgown, holding the top up with what I imagine was either superglue or the same willpower Charlton Heston employs on his loin cloth in Biblical epics, action replays were played on the news to prove that her nipple didn't show on the staircase. It was (sigh of relief) the reflection of the rose she was carrying . . .

Now all we have to worry about is important matters like, is she eating enough, not eating too much, spending too much on clothes? Is she getting blonder, taller, sexier? Is William too fat? Charles getting thin on top? . .

If only Koo Stark were blonde I could type for as long as Norman Mailer.

*W*hat's the good of a dark-haired Princess? Look at Caroline of Monaco. All very well for scandals but simply not the stuff that fairy tales are made of, even in cream silk Valentino and a suntan . . . in fact the suntan is definitely out for the perfect princess.

Even in the days when she was seen in Paris nightclubs with her tits falling out of her dresses when she should have been swotting, Caroline always looked far too abandoned. She was like a beauty from a Gauguin painting. She should have been frolicking up a beach like the boiler at the start of 'Hawaii 5–0', a hibiscus stuck behind one ear. Which is why everyone was so delighted when she went on that rather indiscreet holiday with Guillermo Vilas (an

Argentinian tennis player with gargantuan thighs). Aided only by twenty-foot telephoto lenses, the photographers got shots that proved what *Paris Match* had always suspected . . . Caroline looked in her element wrapped in the surf by Vilas and his thighs, like a latter-day Deborah Kerr with Burt Lancaster in *From Here to Eternity.*

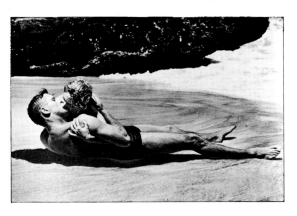

Princess Caroline obviously didn't inherit her mother Grace's serenity, along with not acquiring her icy blondeness. When the utterly-too-beautiful-for-words Grace Kelly met Prince Rainier she was making Hitchcock's eternally stylish film, *To Catch a Thief,* opposite Cary Grant. Hitchcock loved Grace and brought out the best in her, because he saw that underneath all the supposed ice there lay a tumult of such passions that it would take a Cary Grant (at least) to handle her. Grace Kelly was so perfect, such a lady from a good family, that she could get away with kissing him first and still look like she hadn't blinked. Which is rather like she was in real life. Apart from Prince Rainier, with whom she had an almost fairy-tale romance, no one except a real pervert could possibly imagine Grace Kelly DOING IT.

It's like trying to visualize the Pope doing anything racier than singing the odd folk song and kissing the tarmac at airports.

While Grace was in the jungle with Ava Gardner and Clark Gable filming *Mocambo*, it was this facet of her character that was most useful. Ava showered regularly in full view of the native hordes while Grace sat in the shade, a perfect magnolia colour, knitting. But WHO was having the affair with Gable? Naturally everyone imagined it

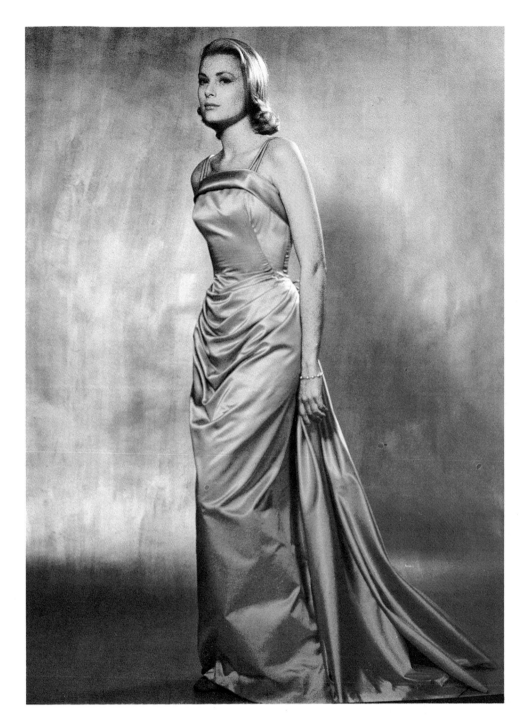

had to be Gardner, Grace was already too revered to be thought of in that light and yet she wasn't pompous or pious, just perfect. Like an orchid.

When Rainier married the orchidous Grace, Monaco was, in the words of Somerset Maugham, 'a sunny spot for shady people'. Grace gave it her all, not just from her wealthy friends and family in Philadelphia, but also with an influx of Hollywood glamour. With the rapier-like business minds of her American associates to assist Rainier in his financial dealings, her influence over him and the future of the Principality was complete.

Princess Grace was cool and infinitely charming in her dealings with everyone involved with or affecting Monaco. She devoted herself to many charitable organizations like the Red Cross, and when she hosted a charitable ball, it had Hollywood glamour as well as regal style.

Princess Grace was the perfect Princess for many people.

And everyone knows who succeeded her as the world's favourite royal blonde . . .

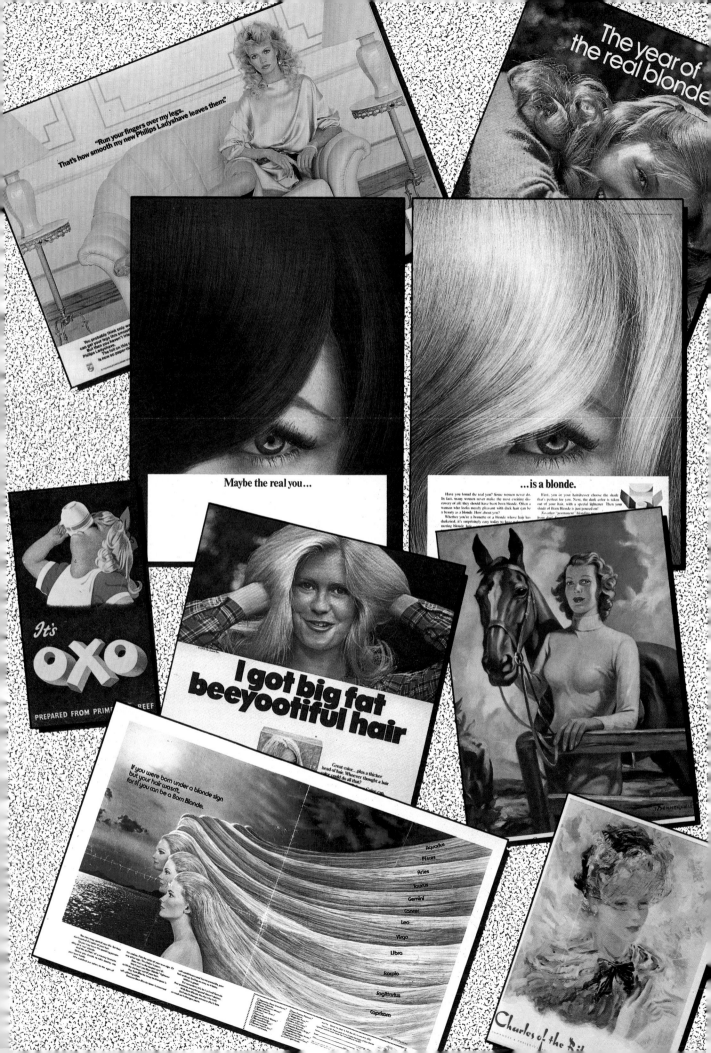

A woman who can't cook for her man isn't all woman

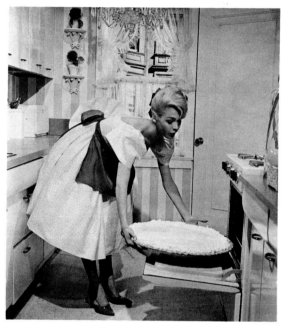

Princess Grace embarked on her career in advertising, with all manner of products. She lent her already regal air and pristine good looks to among other things air freshener (Grace in an apron holding a dish cloth and squirting) and toothpaste. Having a real-life Princess to advertise one's fly sprays and denture creams is an adman's dream, so we should be thankful that Grace's ads are now dated or we might still be seeing them.

In the Forties, pristine blondes in gingham aprons with matching half curtains appeared all over the women's magazines doling out cereal to families of crew-cutted boys. Family life was represented like a set out of 'Leave it to Beaver' without even a sniff of beavers. Mai Britt advertised Lux, who launched their campaign *The World's Most Beautiful Women Use LUX* featuring slightly famous actresses with a splodge of soap on one cheek, who gazed beatifically at the side of the sink. These were not women plagued with husbands who shaved twice a day and left a scum of hairs around the rim of the sink. Their sinks were obviously as clean as their peachy cheeks.

But mainly they were seen in domestic situations. Peering wholesomely into their deep freezes, perching on their colour TVs personifying the American Dream. What seemed to have been forgotten is that blondes were designed to be calculating, manipulative and wear too much lipstick. They were meant to look like Ford Cortinas after a respray, not peer into deep freezes for a leg of lamb. Neither God nor Roger Vadim created blondes to go anywhere near the kitchen.

Any self-respecting blonde is a terrible cook.

Housework is the same. Blondes were put on earth to watch someone else pick the cat hairs off the Wilton. In commercials they're sometimes seen clutching a labour-saving device or surveying the results of a hard day's decorating (like Jilly Cooper for Sanderson) – only you know it's someone else that did the grouting and pasting.

During the Fifties, gingham aprons were flung out of the window. Blondes were accepted as worthy accessories for the successful male and suddenly swathed in mink they were draped across the bonnets of Cadillacs. These bonnets were never less than fourteen blocks long.

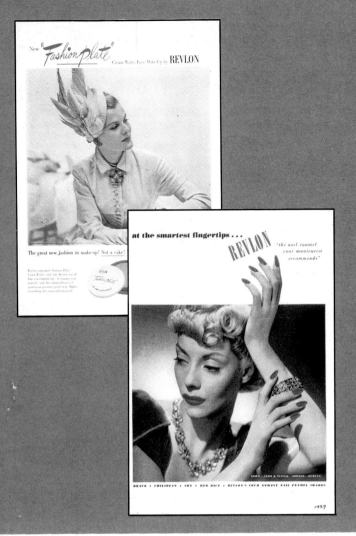

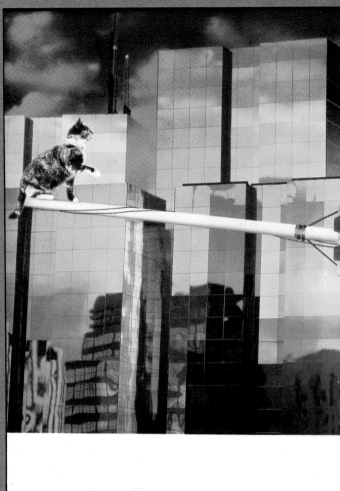

The blonde once and for all has been bound up in Western minds with materialism of all kinds. Especially to Yanks.

But can we trust Americans about anything? I've always felt that it was foolish to trust the judgement of a nation that recently listed petrol, a car, roll-on deodorant and a breath-freshener as the four staples in life they'd most miss.

Since when is Gold Spot a staple? I wonder what these people will do once the apocalypse has deprived them of hash browns, let alone Gold Spot and bidets.

They are obsessed with blondes for the same reason that Europeans were in the Middle Ages. Blondeness to the American symbolizes cleanliness and everyone knows that's next to Godliness.

Tampax is the perfect example of the use of the dual blonde image. First take the youthful athletic ones. This means that youthful would-

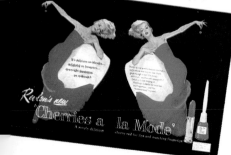

be consumers will image that, while they wait for their braces, pizza faces and terminal cellulite to vanish, they can rival Mark Spitz whenever they get within four feet of water. All that fresh sea air and salty water performing a demabrasion on their spots with only the aid of a Tampax.

The second category has, like the Ugly Duckling, emerged minus any physical imperfections whatsoever. Not wishing to imply that purchasers of their product are damned to a life on the ocean wave, this girl is experiencing life in the fast lane with no punctures. She's the blonde with a red satin bomber jacket with Rich Bitch stamped in glitter on the back. She looks like she's been given the entire contents of the Jackson Five's wardrobe from their '72 tour. She's seen having adventures. She rescues cats off the flagpole on the Empire State Building. It's like *King Kong* and Fay Wray all over again. The cat was probably up there meditating and trying to avoid being photographed for *Interview* magazine again.

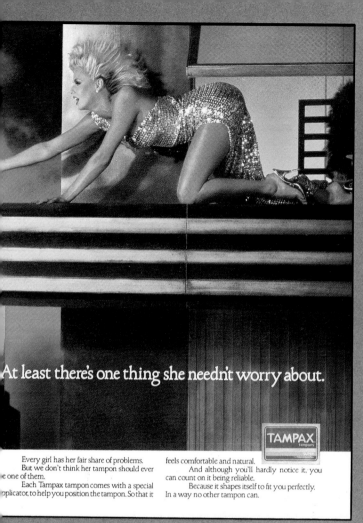

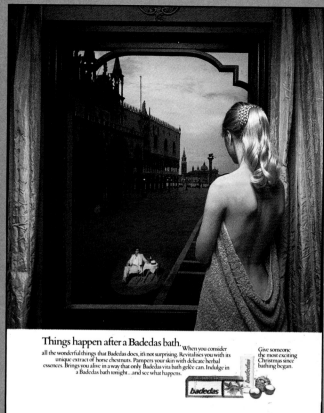

SOME THINGS NEVER CHANGE: another fact utilized by the advertising companies.

As Barbara Cartland has pointed out, all women long to be carried away into the desert by a Sheik. All women except me. I was told at an early age that all Arabs have hereditary syphilis from fucking their camels at times of dire need. I've never recovered from hearing this.

By the same token many women have never got it into their heads that Lancelot was not in fact Franco Nero on a white stallion. So the fantasy of being a trapped beauty about to be rescued from a tall tower continues to be popular.

Now the only difference is that the damsels have had a Badedas bath first...

You know her well. She stands with her back to you in what appears to be the guest bedroom of Vlad the Impaler's castle looking out into the dark starlit night. Either a slavic knight is going to save her or the bloke on skis from the Milk Tray commercial next door but one. There she is without her wimple, blonde and moonlit and Badedas-scented. According to them, 'it's got something to do with the horse chestnuts'. Horse manure. It has something to do with the fact that even from behind with her droopy towel it's patently obvious she has at least a forty-two-inch bust made out of carved alabaster, and you can tell she has the sort of thighs that never look like blancmanges that have been left out in a tropical hailstorm.

Advertisers leave a lot to our imaginations. What does happen after a Badedas bath?

People have believed that if they took enough of a certain vitamin they'd end up as well preserved as Betty Grable. Who can deny that Barbara Cartland looks like a peach in sequins rather than mutton dressed as lamb, but she claims it's all because of the vitamins she takes which include Royal Jelly. I gather this is sweat from the armpits of a Queen Bee and works wonders for the complexion, but in these days of cheap products maybe any sweat will work.

131

Miss Cartland, it is rumoured, assists the effects on her blonde-goddess good looks of these lashings of jelly by always travelling with a lighting man. Of course this may just be vicious lies and conjecture passed around by those other eighty-year-olds less devastating. He lies somewhere under Miss Cartland's chair during TV appearances carefully covered with the hem of her Hartnell pointing a silver foil tray at her chin.

The cleverest bit of association was when one vitamin company used Dinah Shore to advertise their pills at the height of her romance with Burt Reynolds. It wasn't just that Dinah was in her fifties at the time and ravishing, she had Burt as well. What was her secret, we pondered.

Well, *Americans* pondered, as is their wont.

If you ate enough of those vitamins maybe Burt would arrive at your local Women's Institute meeting to display his holiday slides, rounding off the evening with a display of his wall-to-wall pubic hair.

Scent companies know how deeply we long to be someone else. If you can't look like the blonde actress advertising it, at least you can smell like her.

It has to be faced by even the thickest of us that however much we pray at the side of our single beds we are unlikely to wake up as Catherine Deneuve even if we've been drinking Chanel. No matter which pulse spot you've squirted, it ain't gonna work I'm telling you now. But the campaign got everyone squirting like skunks. There she was, that sheaf of heavy golden hair hanging down the side of the glossiest pages in the world, and all I could think was whose faces had she dangled that hair over let alone what did she smell like.

She also looked totally unaware that she was even advertising anything. The best way to look while selling.

Deneuve's image became Chanel's – a welcome improvement. Miss Chanel, it cannot be denied, however talented and innovative she was, had looked like a pekinese with a bad haircut and a lot of gilt jewellery.

Certainly not a person one would wish to smell like. One wants to smell like crumpet not talent.

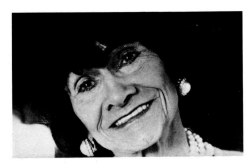

Miss Deneuve on the other hand was PERFECT! Immediately, as you sit in the bath with *Vogue* propped up on your spare tyres you have visions of Catherine, probably trailing a violet mink coat in the mud behind her, having numerous gorgeous children by all manner of ravishing French film stars with unintelligible accents who say things like, 'Geeeve mee your leeps, ma lurve', at the drop of a satin pyjama.

Totally different to the blonde exotic-European appeal of a Deneuve is Farrah Fawcett. I was totally captivated by her advertising campaign for her own shampoo. I could think of nothing nicer than to stand in the shower with Farrah on a rope, all big hair and great big teeth. What an Icon for the Seventies.

Who else made the biggest-selling poster of all time, all because they knew the secret of making their curls subliminally spell out the word S-E-X?

Cary Grant, ahead of Faberge, spotted these unique talents and gave her her own shampoo and conditioner to promote. In keeping with her image: a woman who gargled with TCP, bathed in Dettol and should have spent her entire career wet. The shampoo unfortunately took things one step too far and smelled exactly like a silage farm in very hot weather.

Even having Farrah in the shower with you wasn't enough to combat the indignity of having to walk around for at least a week with a scalp that stank of fertilizer. It was also a tenacious little number. You could easily have played four successive Wimbledon finals with Bjorn Borg and still had a head that smelled like Soylent Green.

No matter what, even now Farrah's cut

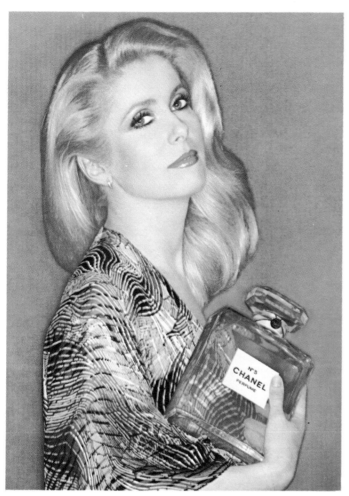

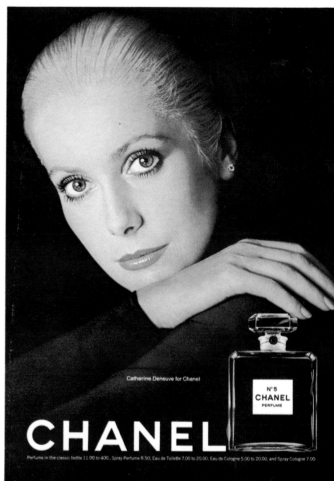

Catherine Deneuve for Chanel

Nº5
CHANEL
PERFUME

CHANEL

Perfume in the classic bottle 11.00 to 400., Spray Perfume 8.50, Eau de Toilette 7.00 to 20.00, Eau de Cologne 5.00 to 20.00, and Spray Cologne 7.00.

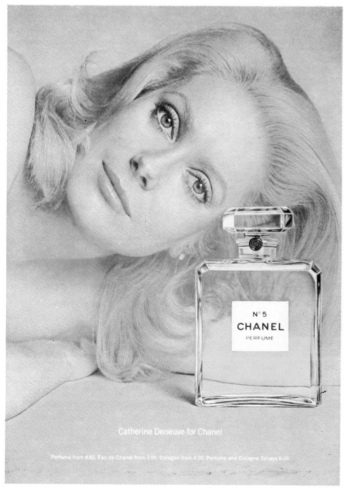

Nº 5
CHANEL
PERFUME

Catherine Deneuve for Chanel

Perfume from 6.50, Eau de Chanel from 7.00, Cologne from 4.00, Perfume and Cologne Sprays 6.00

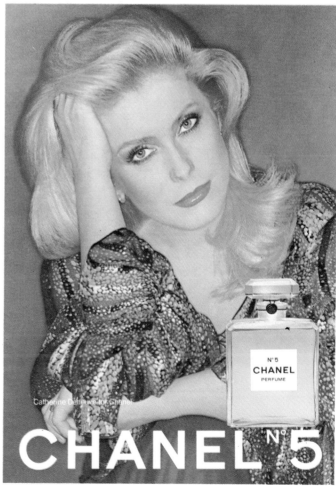

Nº 5
CHANEL
PERFUME

Catherine Deneuve for Chanel

CHANEL Nº 5

all her hair off, I treat my Farrah Fawcett tee shirt like a holy relic. You just can't ever imagine her face downwards on the duvet surrounded by discarded clothes sobbing piteously, I've nothing to wear, you go without me, I wish I'd never been born, etc. She'd be like action woman. Straight on with the Bob Mackie shorts, out on Hollywood Boulevard on her Halston skateboard showing Ryan O'Neal what was what.

But at least having smelled her shampoo I know why she kept flicking her fringe away from her face in every episode of 'Charlie's' whatsits...

Blondes are used a great deal to advertise all manner of unfortunate products in men's magazines. All of these products have the texture of copydex glue, leaving one in some doubt whether you're supposed to glue your erection in place, or whether, with the amount of rubbing it takes to make it sink in, anyone would have a massive stonka. Also they are always called names with racing connotations, like 'Stud' and 'Stally-On'.

In between come things like Sta-Stiff creme and lilac love guns. Why would anyone want a LILAC LOVEGUN?

They also have slogans accompanying the packets – young girls with blonde curly wigs saying 'Will make her shriek', which seems accurate enough, or 'Will make her screw like a bunny.' If these products are so good how come the youthful models on the packets always seem to have had the foresight to borrow a Dynel blonde wig from the local drag show before the photo session?

Blondes also, I have noted in my extensive research, are VERY POPULAR in enema films. For some reason it's considered more erotic to see blondes humiliated. The plots run along the lines, 'Debbie and Tracey wearing virgin white are naughty, chastised severely and then given an enema.' But console yourself with this thought: the dirty old men wanking over these blondes will always be just that, whereas look what an enema a day did for Mae West's complexion.

Last but by no means least we have to include Zsa Zsa Gabor, currently advertising

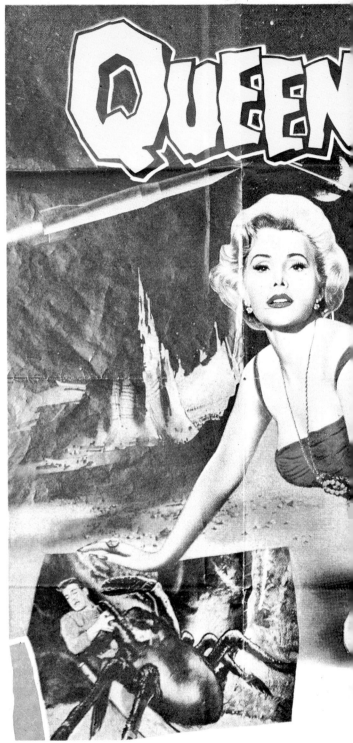

pull-on wigs. She is also about to undergo a lie-detector test, asking the all-important question (for Americans), *Did you marry your husband for money?* The question seems a

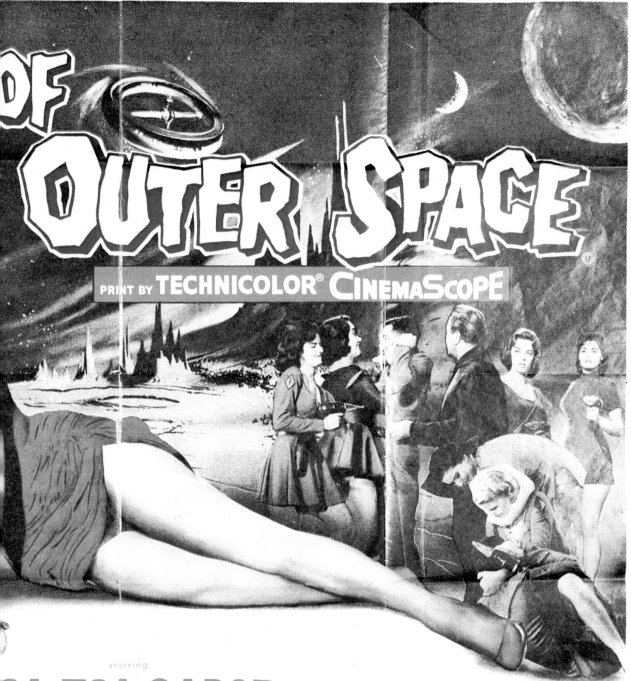

OF OUTER SPACE

PRINT BY TECHNICOLOR® CINEMASCOPE

starring

SA ZSA GABOR ERIC FLEMING · LAURIE MITCHELL · LISA DAVIS

*Zsa Zsa was often heard saying of her husbands, 'OOOOhhh, I luff him, I luff him'.
Miss Gabor could make even pile creams seem like the pinnacle of glamour.*

safe bet for Miss Gabor, who only has to ponder her eight husbands and keep the safest bet's name firmly under her pull-on wig.

Maybe now someone should ask all the celebrities advertising (and they've all been at it for decades) – DID YOU DO IT FOR THE CASH?

135

What actually does happen after a Badedas bath?

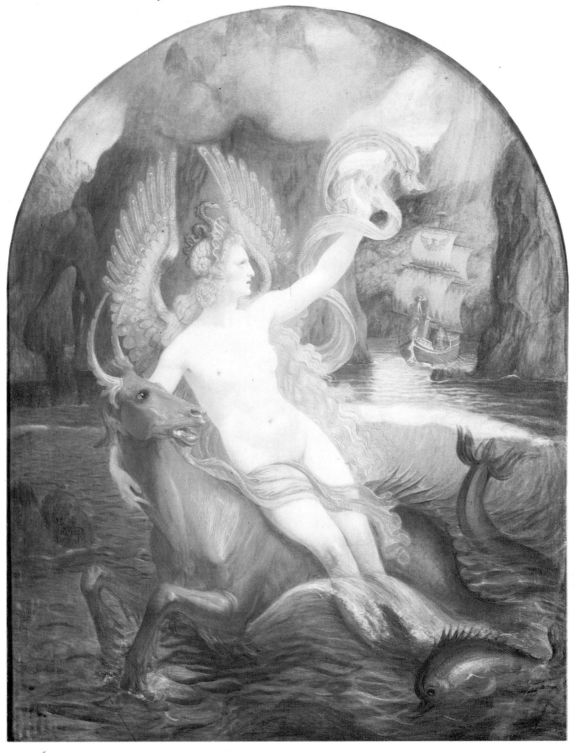

Had advertising companies existed in the Middle Ages they would have had the Sirens lazing on remote rocks exhorting you to lag your pipes, Rapunzel would have been signed on immediately by Clairol, the Ugly Duckling would have found himself doing before-and-after photographs and the Princess with her Pea would have demonstrated the charms of a Slumberland bed.

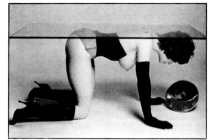

Psychiatrists will tell you that blondes are the most fantasized-about creatures on earth.

Especially if you offer them a small payment to say it.

This has nothing to do with shrinks liking money as much as that along with literary agents, sex symbols and many pop stars, they believe that the true measure of success is a) how many sofas they can cram into their office, b) how long their shagpile is and c) their Alan Jones coffee table.

While you're lying on the sofa shiftily confessing that you thought *The Blue Lagoon* was one of the greatest films ever made, and that you slept with your mother until you were 15, he's merely totting up whether your fee for the past hour will pay for one of those big blondes on all fours with a sheet of plate glass on her back and a patient expression on her face. While you spill the beans he's fantasizing about what exactly he's going to DO on the blonde coffee table once he's fitted his rubber plant, executive toy and ash tray on it. What else will he be able to put on it, he dreams...

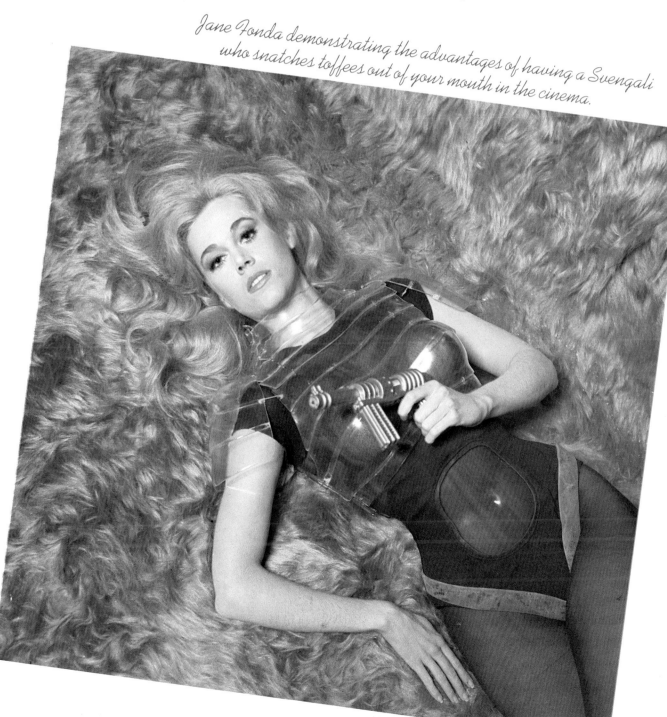

Jane Fonda demonstrating the advantages of having a Svengali who snatches toffees out of your mouth in the cinema.

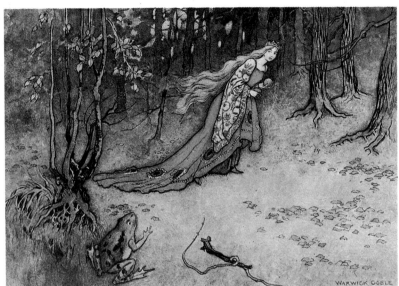

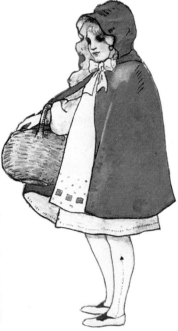

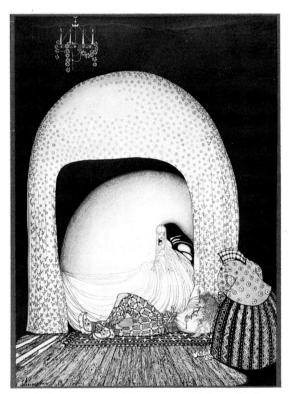

Shrinks have a lot to answer for. Why else would we read so much into what used to be regarded simply as children's fairy tales and charming legends from the fjords, where apart from canoeing there's not a lot else to do except think about blonde princesses trapped in towers of ice. What the modern reader tends to forget is that the frozen tower is not simply some bit of Norwegian whimsy, all their fucking pipes are frozen so why not their towers?

Needless to say, psychiatrists have a field day with the unconscious significance of these stories . . .

All carry a strong message of subliminal sexuality, similar to that of modern advertising. Subliminal in the sense that unless you're a shrink whose living is made by linking everything with cock, you simply wouldn't see it.

Take Lilith. You have to realize that this glorious blonde behaved the way all schoolboys dream their matron's going to until they've actually unpacked their trunk and seen her. She swept into men's bedrooms by magic as they slept and fucked them stupid while they continued to kip on, leaving one in some doubt as to whether the whole experience was that thrilling at all. The guilt of such a smutty dream (or, if it wasn't a dream, the smear of infidelity) was removed by the simple fact that Lilith's golden hair and overpowering sexuality took over entirely.

Lilith got a rough bargain. Although she was transformed in legend from a rampant house matron into almost a demon, doubts were still cast in any cynic's eyes as to her real talents as a seductress by the mere fact that men snored away throughout.

But she became a good explanation for wet dreams.

Had she really been a matron of course, she would have simply been wandering around the corridors at night dispensing

Fairy-tale blondes can feel a pea through twenty-two mattresses.

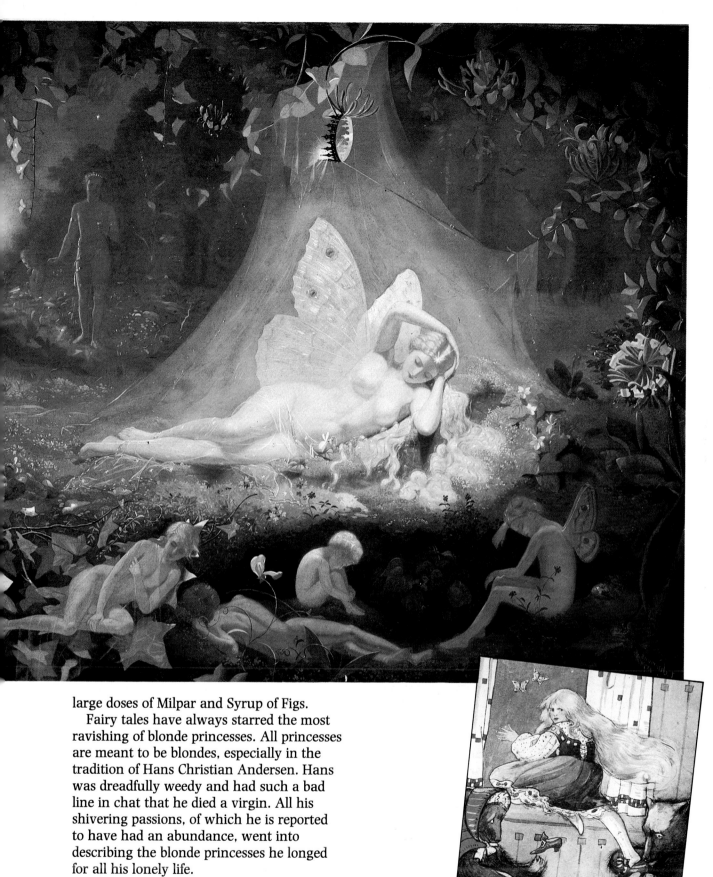

large doses of Milpar and Syrup of Figs.

Fairy tales have always starred the most ravishing of blonde princesses. All princesses are meant to be blondes, especially in the tradition of Hans Christian Andersen. Hans was dreadfully weedy and had such a bad line in chat that he died a virgin. All his shivering passions, of which he is reported to have had an abundance, went into describing the blonde princesses he longed for all his lonely life.

Any psychiatrist worth his salt would have had a FIELD day with Hans.

He displayed his obvious anal fixation when he wrote *The Princess and the Pea*.

SHE·GOT·SUCH· A·FRIGHT·THAT· SHE·BOUNDED· OUT·OF·BED·AND JUMPED·OUT· OF· THE·WINDOW.

Who else would have thought of a tale in which the handsome Prince's one criterion for marriage was that his wife's backside was sensitive enough to feel a pea through twenty-two different mattresses?

The women in *The Little Mermaid* and *The Snow Queen* were all untouchable golden beings, like the women Hans met. He was always longing for a transformation which would give him size three feet and a nose like a pearl button. In *The Ugly Duckling*, even the ugly little grey duckling is transformed at the end into a beautiful big white glistening swan with a wonderful long neck, what more could anyone ask for, even within the boundaries of a fairy tale.

Even poor Rapunzel gets it in the neck from modern psychologists. According to one dissection of this fairy tale it is not just the story of a beautiful princess with golden hair thirty feet long trapped by a wicked king in a tower until a handsome prince comes to save her. The point is that her fair hair overcomes the prince's inhibitions and impotence: his entrance into the tower is a euphemism for his entrance into her body.

Mermaids and the Lorelei had the opposite effect. Instantaneously. Sailors who spotted them basking in the sun, or swimming through the waves splashing their shimmering tails in the sunlight, immediately found themselves steering their ships into the rocks, rather the way a cyclist looking in the window of Lasky's in the Tottenham Court Road inevitably drives into the pavement.

The Lorelei made it even harder for sailors, starved of love and itching from scurvy, to resist. She would sit on a rock overlooking the Rhine combing her hair in an obvious fashion and singing loudly. Sirens initially weren't just hooters attached to ships, they were early mediaeval glamour girls conjured up in the imagination of men who had literally spent years at sea searching for duff places like Lloret de Mar and then thinking they'd found China. While making errors of judgement like this they can be forgiven for thinking they saw and heard mermaids.

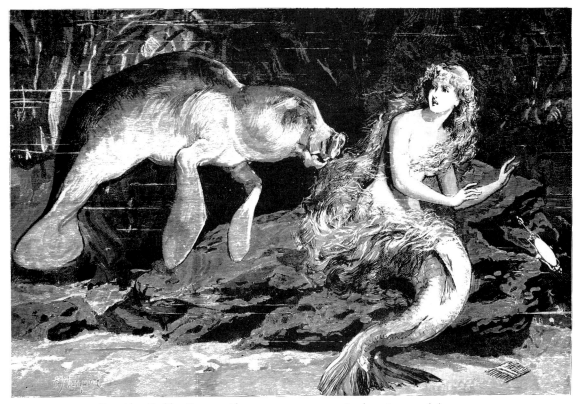

On the Jolly Roger there was a great shortage of lemons.
Long-suffering sailors got scurvy. During high winds they chundered
violently over the side of the boat, only to have it flung
back in their faces. This explains their blurred vision which
led to them mistaking manatees for mermaids.

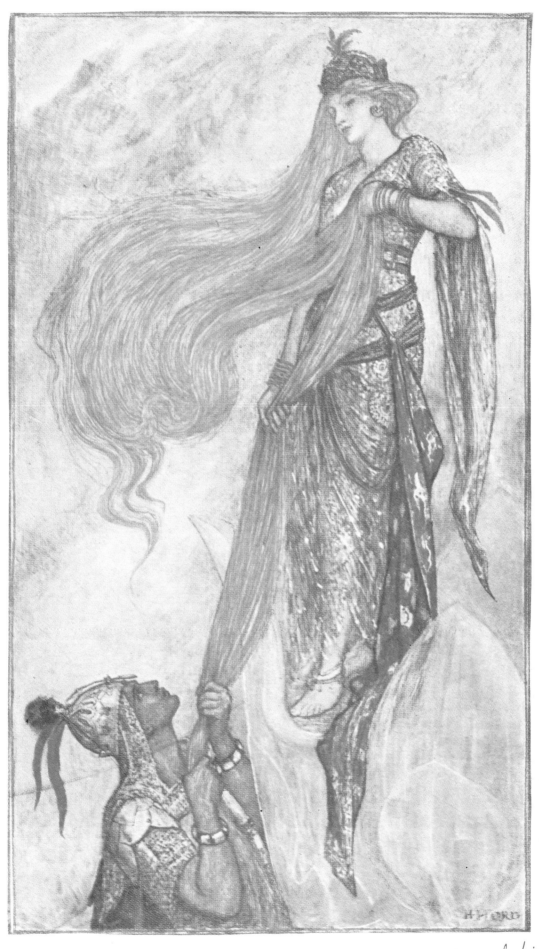

Hold the red, big boys.

Epilogue

inally we must ask the question. What happened to Eve, Adam and the Snake after that fatal bite of the apple?

Basically, the monsoon arrived well ahead of schedule. A crack of thunder swept across the garden and a huge finger shot from out of a gap in the black doom-laden clouds – Adam looked down to where the finger was pointed (probably in derision) and at last he realized that he wasn't wearing his pants. Nor was there anywhere to get a pair as Paki shops weren't open so late then. Mortified and ashamed Adam grabbed a fig leaf and stuck it across his groin.

Theologians tell us that the first miracle was the feeding of the five thousand. They forget about Adam's fig leaf. No one in any painting, sculpture or parchment has ever explained how he held it in position. There are no side straps on his lead, it is unlikely he used cow gum on that sensitive and precious part of his anatomy. No, the fig leaf was a miracle on its own.

Adam hurtled through the garden of Eden, trying to shake off the cockroaches who were trying to crawl up his fig leaf for shelter, as is their wont when the weather gets damp. He understood that he was to be punished eternally and that this was the start of it all.

At the moment of realizing that she was naked too, Eve was lying on her bed surrounded by various leaves trying to decide which one looked best as a going-away outfit from the garden. 'Oh pooh!' she cried, kicking her legs up and down, 'NOTHING looks right on me.' She wondered whether lettuce was too formal or if she should try on a more frilly broccoli style. Around her the thunder cracked ferociously.

And what of the snake who started it all? He too was punished. He slithered out of the garden after Adam and Eve, who had decided to start a market-gardening business. After staying with them as a paying guest for a couple of weeks the snake met his doom in the orchard. He became the first gift that a man ever gave a blonde. The besotted Adam smacked the snake over the head with his hoe and made him into a pair of snakeskin dancing slippers for Eve.

Now in this modern age Eve has come a very long way from being simply a market-gardener's spare rib. Her life and the pleasures she can get from it have increased with each century. Throughout time, blondes have paved the way so that other blondes to follow them will have even more fun.

When you're a blonde you can do anything.

Blondes have become Prime Ministers, have won Nobel Prizes and are now being trained to go to the moon. But as the blonde astronautess is flung into cold water and spun in chambers to simulate weightlessness, what is really on her mind?

How she's going to get a nice pink space suit so that when she has to make that giant step for BLONDEKIND she at least looks good in the photographs.

Nothing stands in your way when you're a blonde except perhaps the wardrobe door. The blonde has come a long long way ...

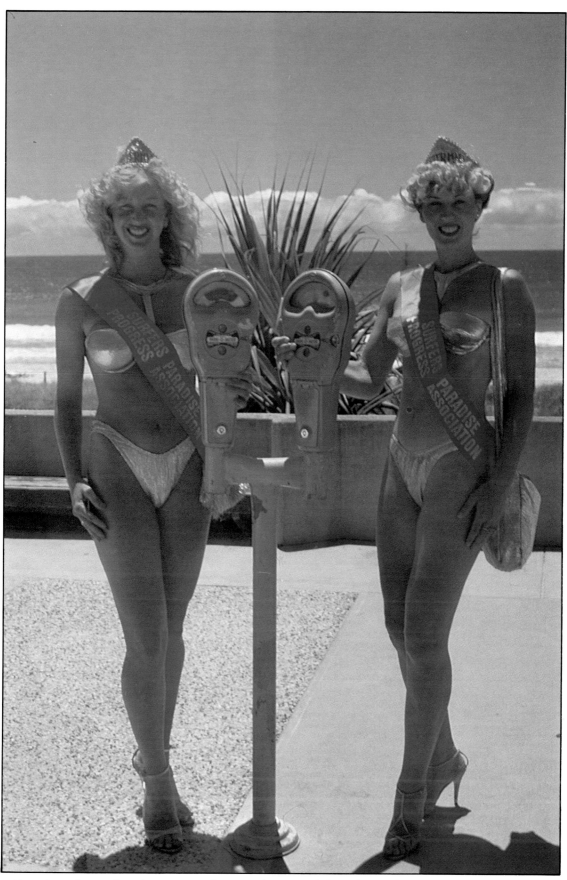

The Garden of Eden may have changed but blondes obviously haven't.

Acknowledgements

I would like to say a special thanks to Sue Ready, who wore a different outfit for every foray into the British Museum, and Bernard Higton, who stayed up late a lot. A big thank you to Philippa Harrison and Ed Victor for their thinly veiled patience and occasional foul moods, their endless inspirational letters. Both of them started out honorary blondes and finished the book grey. I'd like to give Bob, without whom this book would not have been started, a lot of kisses for putting up with several massive wobblers and endless imitations of A. J. P. Taylor.

The illustrations in this book are from the following sources:

Aldus Archive: p.68 *above* (from Mansell Collection), 136, 141,
Brian Aris/Duncan Paul Associates: 119
Aspect Picture Library: 143
Gianni Bozzacchi/Forum: 132
Bridgeman Art Library: 3 *right*, 9 (from Uffizi Gallery, Florence), 10 *bottom left* (from British Museum), 16 *above* (from Roy Miles Fine Paintings), 26 *above* (from Victoria & Albert Museum), 40-1, 70-1 (from Roy Miles Fine Paintings), 138 *below* (from British Library), 139 *above*
BBC Hulton Picture Library: 19, 28, 29 *above* and *below*, 46 *above* and *below*, 47, 48 *above*, 49 *above* 60, 66 *below*, 69 *inset* and *right*, 88 *below*, 97, 122 *bottom left* and *right*
Bulloz (Paris): 56, 65 *inset*
Camera Press: 51, 89, 106
Katherine Cameron: 138 *above right*, 139 *below*
Edimedia: 57 *below* (from National Galleries of Scotland), 67
Mary Evans Picture Library: 10 *above*, 14, 17, 20, 21 *above* and *below*, 24, 25 *centre*, 26 *below*, 27, 42, 43, 45, 48 *below*, 50, 52, 62, 63, 66 *above*, 68 *below*, 72 *above*, 123 *above*, 138 *top left*, 140
Foto Marburg: 37 (hand tinted by Astrid Burchardt)
Adrian George/Francis Kyle Gallery: 5
Burt Glinn/John Hillesdon Agency: 115 *above*
Ronald Grant: 12 *above*, 109 *below*

Philippe Halsman/Magnum: 92, 93, 127
Anwar Hussein: 124
Allen Jones: 137 *above*
Kobal Collection: 10 *below right*, 11, 12 *below right*, 15, 16 *below*, 22 *above* and *below*, 25 *above* and *below*, 53 *inset*, 58, 76-7, 78, 79 (hand tinted by William Taylor), 80 *below*, 81, 84, 85, 86-7, 90-1, 94 *above* and *below*, 96 *above* and *below*, 99, 100, 102 *below*, 108 *right*, 110-11, 112 *above*, 113, 114, 116 *above*, 126, 129, 137 *below*
Kunsthistorisches Museum, Vienna: 13
London Express News and Feature Services: 119 *inset*
Mansell Collection: 32 *above*
Ambrose McEvoy: 73
National Film Archive: 82
National Gallery: 30 *above*
Rex Features: 104-5, 107, 108 *left*, 115 *below*
Royal Pavilion, Brighton: 64-5
Scala/Vision International: 6-7, 31 *above*, 32-3, 38, 39 *above*
Snowdon/Camera Press: 125 *above*
Sotheby's: 34-5
Tate Gallery: 23
John Topham Picture Library: 12 *below left*, 69 *centre*, 88 *above*, 98, 102 *above*, 118 *below left*, 120, 121 *below*, 122 *above*
Universal Pictorial Press: 123 *below*
Wallace Collection: 45, 53, 54-5, 57 *above*
James Wedge/*Cosmopolitan*: 59
Larry Williams/*Observer Magazine*: 34 *inset*

The author and publishers wish to thank the following companies and their advertising agents for their help in supplying material:
Beecham Proprietaries (Badedas), Bristol-Myers (Clairol), Chanel, Philips, Revlon, Tampax Ltd.

Also, thanks to Lady Diana Cooper for her kind permission to use the painting *Called to the Orgy* by Ambrose McEvoy on page 73

Decorated borders by Valerie Hill and Jane Hughes

Front cover photograph by Norman Parkinson for *Tatler*

Picture research by Sue Ready